Essential Best of Five and Multiple Choice Questions for Surgical Finals
Third Edition

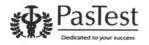
PasTest
Dedicated to your success

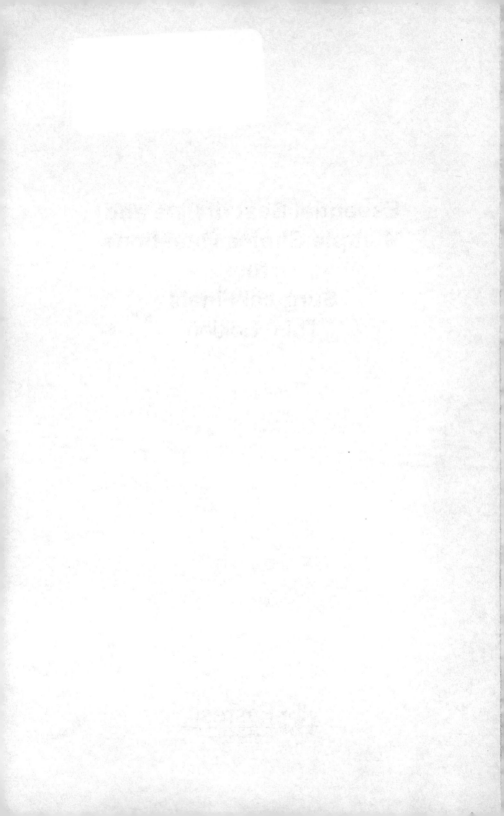

Essential Best of Five and Multiple Choice Questions for Surgical Finals
Third Edition

Delilah Hassanally BSc MBBS MSc FRCS
Consultant Surgeon
Medway Hospital, Kent

Rema Kaur Wasan BA MBBS MA MRCP FRCR
Consultant Radiologist
King's College Hospital, London

Shahzad G Raja BSc MBBS MRCS
Specialist Registrar Cardiothoracic Surgery
Western Infirmary, Glasgow

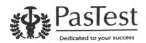
PasTest
Dedicated to your success

© 2007 PASTEST LTD
Egerton Court
Parkgate Estate
Knutsford
Cheshire
WA16 8DX

Telephone: 01565 752000

First published 1997
Reprinted 1999, 2001, 2003
Second edition 2003
Third edition 2007

ISBN 1 904627 81 1
ISBN 978 1 904627 814

A catalogue record for this book is available from the British Library.

The information contained within this book was obtained by the authors from reliable sources. However, while every effort has been made to ensure its accuracy, no responsi-bility for loss, damage or injury occasioned to any person acting or refraining from action as a result of information contained herein can be accepted by the publishers or authors.

PasTest Revision Books and Intensive Courses

PasTest has been established in the field of postgraduate medical education since 1972, providing revision books and intensive study courses for doctors preparing for their professional examinations. Books and courses are available for the following specialties:

MRCP Part 1 and Part 2, MRCPCH Part 1 and Part 2, MRCS, MRCOG, MRCGP, DRCOG, MRCPsych, DCH, FRCA and PLAB.

For further details contact:

PasTest, Freepost, Knutsford, Cheshire WA16 7BR

Tel: 01565 752000 Fax: 01565 650264

E-mail: enquiries@pastest.co.uk

Web site: www.pastest.co.uk

Typeset by Saxon Graphics Ltd, Derby
Printed and bound by Cambridge University Press, Cambridge

CONTENTS

INTRODUCTION

There are now many multiple choice question books for both under-graduate and postgraduate medical examinations. The aim of this book is to provide 'real'-type practice examinations at the appropriate level for under-graduates sitting their final surgical examinations. These questions will also benefit those sitting the PLAB examination.

This book contains four test papers designed to be similar in format, content and balance of subjects to surgical finals examinations. Answers and detailed teaching notes are given for each question. The questions are as 'real' as possible – they include material that has been remembered over the years by medical students after their surgical finals examinations. They also include the new-style 'Best of five' questions, which themselves pose a different style of examination.

There is a natural tendency to recall the harder and more confusing topics, but, rather than avoiding these, we have deliberately included them and so the pass mark for each paper is probably a little less than 50%. We hope medical students will use this to their advantage; everyone will get the easy questions right, but the medical student who enters the examination having done the more difficult questions should not just pass, but pass well.

We are delighted to include within this third edition a new range of best of five MCQs, included in each paper. This is to reflect the changes and recent developments in the types of questions met at both undergraduate and postgraduate level. In addition, we have reviewed all the questions and answers and made appropriate changes to maintain current medical opinion.

MCQ EXAMINATION TECHNIQUE

Before sitting an MCQ examination, you will need to know how many questions are likely to be on the paper and how long you will be given to complete it. Thus you will be able to assess the approximate amount of time that can be spent on each question. Pacing yourself accurately during the examination to finish on time, or with time to spare, is essential.

In MCQ examinations you must read the question (both stem and items A–E) carefully. Take care not to mark the wrong boxes and think very carefully before making a mark on the answer sheet. There are two types of MCQs: True/False and Best of Five. Both are featured in each of the four exam papers in this book.

For True/False MCQ's regard each item as being independent of every other item – each refers to a specific quantum of knowledge. The item (or the stem and the item taken together) make up a statement for True/False MCQs. You are required to indicate whether you regard this statement as 'true' or 'false'. You must answer each stem. Look only at a single statement when answering – disregard all the other statements presented in the question. They have nothing to do with the item you are concentrating on.

The technique of approaching Best of Five MCQs is different. Remember that as the answer is the 'best of five' all five stems offered must be analyzed. Consider all the details in the stem – usually a clinical scenario. Look for clues. Fish out the red herrings. Try to think of the answer before viewing the stems. That way if your answer is included in the stems you will be a winner! More than one stem can be correct – it is the MOST correct which is right. One will frequently find it easy to narrow down the answers to two stems. The challenge is making the final correct decision.

Good luck from us all.

As you go through the questions, you can either mark your answers immediately on the answer sheet or you can mark them on the question paper and then transfer them to the answer sheet. If you adopt the second approach you must take great care not to make any errors and not to run out of time, since you will not be allowed extra time to transfer marks to the answer sheet. The answer sheet must always be marked neatly and carefully according to the instructions given. Careless marking is probably one of the commonest causes of rejection of answer sheets by the document reader.

- Do as many good quality practice papers as possible. This will help you to identify your strengths and weaknesses in time for further study. You can also use the Revision Index at the back of this book to find questions on specific topics, so that after you have done some reading you can test your knowledge.

- With the four exams provided in this book be strict with yourself and work under realistic exam conditions. You should develop an understanding of your own work rate so that you know how much time you can spend on each question.

- Read each question several times. Nobody at this vital stage in their career should be wasting marks because they misread or misunderstood the question.

- Each exam in this book contains 60 questions (15 Best of Five and 45 True/False Questions).

- If you have to guess the answer to a question, put a special mark next to it. You will then be able to find out if you are a good guesser. This is especially important if your examination is negatively marked, i.e. marks will be deducted for incorrect answers. It is important to know what you know as well as what you don't know.

- Use the Revision Checklist on the following pages to keep a record of the subjects you have covered and feel confident about. This will ensure that you do not miss out any key topics.

SAMPLE ANSWER SHEET

UNIVERSITY OF LONDON Management Systems Division

MULTIPLE-CHOICE EXAMINATION ANSWER SHEET

DATE...

SURNAME...

FIRST NAME(S)...

Instructions: Use the HB pencil provided. To make an answer draw a single horizontal line along the dotted line above the appropriate letter or number. To answer 'TRUE' draw your line above the capital letter in the upper row. To answer 'FALSE' draw your line above the lower case letter in the lower row. For example:

[A] for 'TRUE'   [A] for 'FALSE'
[a]   [a]

If you change your mind and wish to cancel a completed answer, draw another line below the letter or number, along the dotted line. Do not rub out.

Candidate No.	Test No.	College No.
[0] [0] [0] [0]	[0] [0] [0] [0]	[0] [0]
[1] [1] [1] [1]	[1] [1] [1] [1]	[1] [1]
[2] [2] [2] [2]	[P] [2] [2] [2]	[2] [2]
[3] [3] [3] [3]	[3] [3] [3]	[3] [3]
[4] [4] [4] [4]	[4] [4] [4]	[4] [4]
[5] [5] [5] [5]	[5] [5] [5]	[5] [5]
[6] [6] [6] [6]	[6] [6] [6]	[6] [6]
[7] [7] [7] [7]	[7] [7] [7]	[7] [7]
[8] [8] [8] [8]	[8] [8] [8]	[8] [8]
[9] [9] [9] [9]	[9] [9] [9]	[9] [9]

Shown below is the correct method of completion, the correct method of cancellation/alteration and examples of various incorrect methods of completion.

CORRECT METHOD OF COMPLETION

True = [A]   False = [A]
       [a]   [a]

CORRECT METHOD OF CANCELLATION/ALTERATION

To cancel a response, draw a line below the letter. Do not rub out. Thus:

[A] or [A] = Cancelled
[a]   [a]

To alter a response, first cancel. Then draw a line above the other letter. Thus:

False = [A]   True = [A]
        [a]   [a]

INCORRECT METHODS OF COMPLETION

Too faint   [A]
Slanted   [A]
Too low   [A]
Too high   [A]
Into next box   [A] [B]
Too short   [A] [A] [A]
Isolated cancellation [A]
DETERMINATE TYPE T

1	A B C D E / a b c d e	13 A B C D E / a b c d e	25 A B C D E / a b c d e	37 A B C D E / a b c d e	49 A B C D E / a b c d e
2	A B C D E / a b c d e	14 A B C D E / a b c d e	26 A B C D E / a b c d e	38 A B C D E / a b c d e	50 A B C D E / a b c d e
3	A B C D E / a b c d e	15 A B C D E / a b c d e	27 A B C D E / a b c d e	39 A B C D E / a b c d e	51 A B C D E / a b c d e
4	A B C D E / a b c d e	16 A B C D E / a b c d e	28 A B C D E / a b c d e	40 A B C D E / a b c d e	52 A B C D E / a b c d e
5	A B C D E / a b c d e	17 A B C D E / a b c d e	29 A B C D E / a b c d e	41 A B C D E / a b c d e	53 A B C D E / a b c d e
6	A B C D E / a b c d e	18 A B C D E / a b c d e	30 A B C D E / a b c d e	42 A B C D E / a b c d e	54 A B C D E / a b c d e
7	A B C D E / a b c d e	19 A B C D E / a b c d e	31 A B C D E / a b c d e	43 A B C D E / a b c d e	55 A B C D E / a b c d e
8	A B C D E / a b c d e	20 A B C D E / a b c d e	32 A B C D E / a b c d e	44 A B C D E / a b c d e	56 A B C D E / a b c d e
9	A B C D E / a b c d e	21 A B C D E / a b c d e	33 A B C D E / a b c d e	45 A B C D E / a b c d e	57 A B C D E / a b c d e
10	A B C D E / a b c d e	22 A B C D E / a b c d e	34 A B C D E / a b c d e	46 A B C D E / a b c d e	58 A B C D E / a b c d e
11	A B C D E / a b c d e	23 A B C D E / a b c d e	35 A B C D E / a b c d e	47 A B C D E / a b c d e	59 A B C D E / a b c d e
12	A B C D E / a b c d e	24 A B C D E / a b c d e	36 A B C D E / a b c d e	48 A B C D E / a b c d e	60 A B C D E / a b c d e

Reproduced by kind permission of the University of London.

REVISION CHECKLIST

Use this checklist to record your revision progress. Tick the subjects when you feel confident that you have covered them adequately. This will ensure that you do not forget to revise any key topics. This list is arranged in approximate order of importance. Items closest to the top of each list are most likely to come up in examinations.

GASTROINTESTINAL SYSTEM – UPPER
- [ ] Acid reflux
- [ ] Peptic ulcer
- [ ] Achalasia
- [ ] Upper gastrointestinal bleed
- [ ] Small bowel obstruction
- [ ] Mesenteric embolus
- [ ] Crohn's disease
- [ ] Post-gastrectomy symptoms
- [ ] Oesophageal malignancy
- [ ] Paralytic ileus
- [ ] Pancreatitis; pancreatic tumours
- [ ] Acute appendicitis
- [ ] Hernias – femoral and inguinal
- [ ] Parotid tumours
- [ ] Carcinoma of the tongue
- [ ] Barium studies; endoscopy

GASTROINTESTINAL SYSTEM – LOWER
- [ ] Inflammatory bowel disease
- [ ] Diverticular disease
- [ ] Malignancy
- [ ] Fistulae
- [ ] Haemorrhoids
- [ ] Anal fissure
- [ ] Pilonidal abscess

HEPATOBILIARY SYSTEM
- [ ] Gallstones
- [ ] Cholecystitis
- [ ] Ascending cholangitis

❏ Jaundice
❏ Radiological procedures, eg ERCP (endoscopic retrograde
        cholangiopancreatography), PTC (percutaneous transhepatic
        cholangiogram)
❏ Hepatitis B
❏ Hydatid cyst of the liver

VASCULAR
Venous
❏ Varicose veins
❏ Deep vein thrombosis
Arterial
❏ Ischaemia
❏ Carotid stenosis
❏ Peripheral vascular disease

RENAL SYSTEM
❏ Neoplasia
❏ Calculi
❏ Acute renal failure
❏ Investigations, eg intravenous urography

UROGENITAL TRACT
❏ Testicular tumours
❏ Scrotal swellings
❏ Varicocele
❏ Hydrocele
❏ Undescended testes

TRAUMA
❏ Chest
❏ Spleen
❏ Kidney
❏ Head

SKIN
❏ Malignant melanoma
❏ Carbuncle
❏ Basal cell carcinoma

NERVOUS SYSTEM
❏ Horner syndrome
❏ Bell's palsy

MISCELLANEOUS
❏ Breast – benign and malignant lesions
❏ Thyroid – cystic and solid swellings
❏ Postoperative complications
❏ Wound healing
❏ Fluid replacement
❏ Shock/hypovolaemia

OPERATIONS CHECKLIST
Medical students need to be aware of certain operations that are performed routinely. This short list is by no means comprehensive, but can be used as a guideline. You need to know the indication for the operation and basic principles about pre- and postoperative management. There is no need for detailed knowledge on the procedure itself. Use this list to tick off the procedures when you feel confident of your knowledge.

GASTROINTESTINAL TRACT
❏ Oesophagectomy
❏ Billroth I and Billroth II (polya) gastrectomy
❏ Small bowel resection
❏ Appendicectomy
❏ Hemicolectomy, subtotal colectomy, stomas
❏ Hartmann's procedure
❏ Anterior resection and abdominoperineal resection of the rectum
❏ Haemorrhoidectomy
❏ Lateral sphincterotomy

VASCULAR
❏ Carotid endarterectomy
❏ Femoral–popliteal artery bypass graft
❏ High saphenous ligation and stripping of the long saphenous vein

BREAST
❏ Lumpectomy
❏ Mastectomy

THYROID
❏ Lobectomy, total thyroidectomy

UROLOGY
❏ Transurethral resection of the prostate (TURP)
❏ Nephrectomy

OTHERS
❏ Laparoscopic cholecystectomy
❏ Lichtenstein's repair of inguinal hernias
❏ Nissen's fundoplication for hiatus hernia
❏ Incision and drainage of abscess

ABBREVIATIONS

ACTH	adrenocorticotrophic hormone
ADH	antidiuretic hormone
A&E	accident and emergency
AIDS	acquired immune deficiency syndrome
APTT	activated partial thromboplastin time
ARDS	acute respiratory distress syndrome
BMI	body mass index
BP	blood pressure
CMV	cytomegalovirus
CPA	cyproterone acetate
CREST	calcinosis, Raynaud's phenomenon, (o)esophageal dysfunction, sclerodactyly and telangiectasia
CSF	cerebrospinal fluid
CT	computed tomography
CT-KUB	computed tomography of the kidney, ureter and bladder
CTS	carpal tunnel syndrome
CVP	central venous pressure
DIC	disseminated intravascular coagulation
DNA	deoxyribonucleic acid
DVT	deep vein thrombosis
EBV	Epstein–Barr virus
ECG	electrocardiogram
ERCP	endoscopic retrograde cholangiopancreatography
ESR	erythrocyte sedimentation rate
FAP	familial adenomatous polyposis
FBC	full blood count
FT_4	free thyroxine
GA	general anaesthesia
GCS	Glasgow Coma Scale
GI	gastrointestinal
GOJ	gastro-oesophageal junction
H^+	hydrogen ion
β-hCG	β human chorionic gonadotrophin
HIV	human immunodeficiency virus
HNPCC	hereditary non-polyposis colon cancer
5HT	5–hydroxytryptamine or serotonin
HTLV	human T-cell lymphotrophic virus
HVA	homovanillic acid
ICU	intensive care unit

INR	international normalised ratio
IU	international units
IVC	inferior vena cava
IVU	intravenous urography
LFTs	liver function tests
LHRH	luteinising hormone-releasing hormone
LMP	last menstrual period
MRI	magnetic resonance imaging
NGT	nasogastric tube
NSAID	non-steroidal anti-inflammatory drug
Pco_2	partial pressure of carbon dioxide
PE	pulmonary embolus
PEG	percutaneous endoscopic gastrostomy
PSA	prostate-specific antigen
PT	prothrombin time
PTC	percutaneous transhepatic cholangiography
RIF	right iliac fossa
RNA	ribonucleic acid
RLN	recurrent laryngeal nerve
RTA	road traffic accident
T_4	thyroxine
TB	tuberculosis
TPN	total parenteral nutrition
TSH	thyroid-stimulating hormone
U&Es	urea and electrolytes
UTI	urinary tract infection
VATER	vertebral, anorectal, tracheoesophageal, renal or radial anomalies
VMA	vanillylmandelic acid
WCC	white cell count

NORMAL RANGES

Serum	Normal range
Albumin	36–52 g/L
Amylase	70–300 IU/L
Bicarbonate	22–28 mmol/L
Bilirubin	5–20 μmol/L
Calcium	2.20–2.60 mmol/L
Chloride	95–105 mmol/L
Creatinine kinase	23–175 IU/L
Creatinine	60–120 μmol/L
γ-Glutamyl transferase (GGT)	< 40 IU/L
Globulins	24–37 g/L
Immunoglobulins	
IgG	5.3–16.5 g/L
IgA	0.8–4.0 g/L
IgM	0.5–2.0 g/L
Iron	14–29 μmol/L
Total iron-binding capacity (TIBC)	45–75 μmol/L
Lactate dehydrogenase (LDH)	100–300 IU/L
Magnesium	0.70–1.00 mmol/L
Osmolarity	270–295 mosmol/L
Phosphatase (acid)	0–4 IU/L
Phosphatase (alkaline)	40–115 IU/L
Phosphate	0.8–1.4 mmol/L
Potassium	3.5–5.0 mmol/L
Protein	62–82 g/L
Sodium	135–145 mmol/L
Thyroid function tests	
T_4	54–144 nmol/L
TSH	0.10–5.0 mU/L
Triiodothyronine (T_3)	0.8–2.7 nmol/L
FT_4	9–25 pmol/L
Thyroxine-binding globulin	10–30 mg/L
Transaminase ALT	11–55 IU/L
Transaminase AST	13–42 IU/L
Transferrin	2–4 g/L
Urate	0.24–0.45 mmol/L
Urea	2.5–6.6 mmol/L

Plasma

Glucose	3.0–5.9 mmol/L
Arterial blood gases	
H^+	36–43 nmol/L
Pco_2	4.6–6.0 kPa
Bicarbonate	20–28 mmol/L
Po_2	10.5–13.5 kPa
Lactate	0.63–2.44 mmol/L
Pyruvate	34–80 µmol/L

Cerebrospinal fluid (CSF)

Glucose	2.5–3.9 mmol/L
Protein	< 0.45 g/L

Urine

Catecholamines	< 1.3 µmol/24 h
VMA (HMMA)	9–36 µmol/24 h
5HIAA	10–50 µmol/24 h
Microalbumin	< 30 mg/L
Creatinine clearance	60–110 ml/min

Miscellaneous

Faecal fat	< 10 mmol/24h
Xylose excretion test	
Urine excretion (25g dose)	> 33 mmol/5 h
Urine excretion (5 g dose)	> 8 mmol/5 h
Blood xylose at 1 h (25 g dose)	2.0–4.8 mmol/L
Blood xylose at 2 h (25g dose)	1.0–5.0 mmol/L

BEST OF FIVE AND MULTIPLE CHOICE QUESTIONS PAPER 1

60 questions: time allowed 2½ hours

Best of Five Questions
Mark your answers with a tick (True) in the box provided.

1.1 A 65-year-old man was brought to A&E with sudden onset of severe back pain lasting 20 minutes. The pain was constant and not exacerbated by coughing or sneezing. On examination the patient was in shock with a palpable 8 cm mass deep in the epigastrium above the umbilicus. His past history suggested a 6 cm abdominal aortic aneurysm diagnosed 2 years ago at the time of cholecystectomy. The patient is a non-smoker and drinks 2 pints of beer a week. This patient most probably has:

- ☐ A Acute cholecystitis
- ☐ B Acute pancreatitis
- ☐ C Herniated lumbar disc
- ☐ D Acute appendicitis
- ☐ E Rupturing abdominal aortic aneurysm

1.2 A house surgeon performing his first appendicectomy was unable to identify the base of the appendix as a result of massive adhesions in the peritoneal cavity. The consultant suggested to him identifying the caecum first and then localising the base of the appendix. What anatomical structure(s) on the caecum would he have used to find the base of the appendix?

- ☐ A Omental appendages
- ☐ B Haustra coli
- ☐ C Ileal orifice
- ☐ D Semilunar folds
- ☐ E Taeniae coli

1.3 A 50–year-old man with severe ureteric colic has an impacted 8 mm stone at the pelviureteric junction. He has an unremarkable past medical history and his laboratory investigations are normal. Which of the following will be the most appropriate management strategy for this patient?

☐ A Extracorporeal shock wave lithotripsy
☐ B Endoscopic retrograde basket extraction
☐ C Endoscopic retrograde laser vaporisation of the stone
☐ D Open surgical removal
☐ E Waiting for spontaneous passage of stone

1.4 A 23-year-old typist has signs and symptoms of carpal tunnel syndrome. These clinical features always result from compression of what structure in the carpal tunnel?

☐ A Median nerve
☐ B Radial artery
☐ C Superficial radial nerve
☐ D Ulnar artery
☐ E Ulnar nerve

1.5 A 65-year-old man presents in A&E with abdominal distension, diffuse mild tenderness and hyperactive bowel sounds in the mid-abdomen. He had undergone right hemicolectomy for a 2 cm malignant polyp in the ascending colon 6 weeks ago. An erect abdominal radiograph shows multiple air fluid levels in the small intestine. What is the next most appropriate step in management?

☐ A Abdominal computed tomography (CT)
☐ B Barium enema
☐ C Small bowel series
☐ D Placement of nasogastric tube
☐ E Surgical exploration

1.6 A previously healthy 80-year-old woman is hospitalised for surgery to replace the broken hip that she sustained as a result of fall down stairs, and is then moved to a nursing home; however, she is unable to ambulate until about a month later, when she dies suddenly. Which of the following is most likely to be the immediate cause of death found at postmortem examination?

- A Tuberculosis (TB)
- B Pulmonary embolism
- C Pneumonia with pneumococcus
- D Congestive heart failure
- E Carcinoma of the uterus

1.7 **A 50-year-old man has experienced pain with urination for the past week. His temperature is 37.5°C. On digital rectal examination his prostate is slightly enlarged and mildly tender to palpation. Laboratory studies show his white blood cell count (WCC) to be 13 000/mm³. Urine culture grows > 100 000 *Escherichia coli* organisms. His serum prostate-specific antigen (PSA) is 6 ng/mL. He receives antibiotic therapy and improves. This condition recurs six times in the next 12 months. What is the most likely diagnosis for this patient?**

- A Nodular prostatic hyperplasia
- B Prostatic adenocarcinoma
- C Chronic bacterial prostatitis
- D Prostodynia
- E Urothelial carcinoma of urethra

1.8 **A 50-year-old woman underwent a total thyroidectomy for follicular carcinoma of the thyroid gland. Within a day of surgery, she is noted to have tingling sensations and neuromuscular irritability. Which of the following serum laboratory tests should be ordered immediately to determine further therapy for this woman?**

- A Calcitonin
- B TSH (thyroid-stimulating hormone)
- C Total thyroxine (T_4)
- D Ionised calcium
- E Parathyroid hormone

1.9 A male infant, on physical examination immediately after birth, is noticed to have an abnormal opening of the urethra on to the ventral surface of the penis for a distance of 0.3 cm. Which of the following is the most probable diagnosis?

- ❏ A Cryptorchidism
- ❏ B Exstrophy
- ❏ C Hypospadias
- ❏ d Epispadias
- ❏ E Phimosis

1.10 A 75-year-old woman presents with severe left lower quadrant abdominal pain lasting 10 hours. She is known to have chronic constipation. On examination her temperature is 39.2°C and there is tenderness and guarding in the left iliac fossa. An erect abdominal radiograph shows free air under the diaphragm. This patient most probably has:

- ❏ A Crohn's disease
- ❏ B Perforation of a colonic diverticulum
- ❏ C Hirschsprung's disease
- ❏ D Appendicitis
- ❏ E Pancreatitis

1.11 A 45-year-old obese patient, on postoperative day 2 after gastric bypass operation for weight reduction, complains of sudden onset of severe right-sided chest pain accompanied by tachypnoea, tachycardia and desaturation. The pain is pleuritic in origin. Which of the following is the most appropriate diagnostic investigation for this patient?

- ❏ A CT
- ❏ B MRI (magnetic resonance imaging)
- ❏ C ECG
- ❏ D Chest radiograph
- ❏ E Ventilation–perfusion scan

1.12 A 25-year-old man is brought to A&E after a bar fight in which he was stabbed in the right chest. On arrival he was haemodynamically stable, with reduced air entry on the right side of his chest. His oxygen saturation on room air was 90%. A chest radiograph showed a haemopneumothorax on the affected side. What is the next most appropriate step in his management?

- [ ] A   Masterly inactivity
- [ ] B   Endotracheal intubation and mechanical ventilation
- [ ] C   Prescription of antibiotics
- [ ] D   Insertion of a chest drain
- [ ] E   Exploratory thoracotomy

1.13 A 50-year-old man with progressively increasing anaemia was found to have positive faecal occult blood. On further enquiry he revealed that his bowel habits have changed over the last few months. On physical examination he was pale and dyspnoeic, but otherwise his examination was unremarkable. Laboratory investigations suggested iron deficiency anaemia. Which of the following will be the most appropriate investigation to establish diagnosis in this patient?

- [ ] A   Abdominal angiography
- [ ] B   Abdominal radiograph
- [ ] C   Barium swallow
- [ ] D   Colonoscopy
- [ ] E   Upper gastrointestinal endoscopy

1.14 A 32-year-old stockbroker has developed difficulty in swallowing solids over the last few months, with no problem swallowing liquids. He is a non-smoker and denies any alcohol use. There is nothing significant in his past medical history except that he has been using antacids and H_2-receptor blockers for gastro-oesophageal reflux disease for the last 5 years with limited symptomatic relief. His clinical examination is normal. What is the most likely cause of this man's dysphagia?

- [ ] A   Diffuse oesophageal spasm
- [ ] B   Lower oesophageal web
- [ ] C   Oesophageal squamous carcinoma
- [ ] D   Scleroderma
- [ ] E   Peptic oesophageal stricture

1.15 A 20-year-old victim of a high-speed car collision had a right-sided pneumothorax, along with fracture of the pelvic and right humerus. A chest drain was inserted, which kept on bubbling over the next few days. The air leak got worse when the drain was connected to low-grade suction and the lung failed to expand fully. What is the most likely cause of this complication?

- [ ] A Air embolism
- [ ] B Oesophageal injury
- [ ] C Injury to major bronchus
- [ ] D Tension pneumothorax
- [ ] E Fat embolism

Multiple Choice Questions

Mark your answers with a tick (True) or a cross (False) in the box provided. Leave the box blank for 'Don't know'. Do not look at the answers until you have completed the whole question paper.

1.16   In the management of a patient with a head injury:

- ❑ A   The airway is not a problem
- ❑ B   A raised blood pressure (eg 190/100 mmHg) with bradycardia suggests hypovolaemia
- ❑ C   A patient who is making groaning sounds with eyes spontaneously open and localising pain has a Glasgow Coma Scale (GCS) score of 11
- ❑ D   A CT scan is mandatory
- ❑ E   A helmet should not be removed

1.17   Acute appendicitis:

- ❑ A   Causes pain in the umbilical area, which 'moves' to the right iliac fossa (RIF)
- ❑ B   Can be excluded if the WCC and temperature are normal
- ❑ C   Can be mistaken for ovarian cyst rupture
- ❑ D   Can be treated by laparoscopic appendicectomy
- ❑ E   Mimics mesenteric adenitis

1.18   A chest drain:

- ❑ A   Is essential for the treatment of pneumothorax
- ❑ B   Is inserted under general anaesthetic
- ❑ C   Is essential for the treatment of tension pneumothorax
- ❑ D   Is inserted for drainage of empyema
- ❑ E   Can be used to drain a haemothorax

1.19   Clinical features of hyperthyroidism include:

- ❑ A   Atrial fibrillation
- ❑ B   Weight loss
- ❑ C   Bradycardia
- ❑ D   Intolerance to cold
- ❑ E   Exophthalmos

1.20   Clinical features of prolapsed intervertebral disc at the L5–S1 level include:

- ❏ A   Back pain
- ❏ B   Pain on straight-leg raising
- ❏ C   Absence of the knee jerk
- ❏ D   Loss of sensation on the outer border of the foot
- ❏ E   Weakness of foot inversion

1.21   Carpal tunnel syndrome (CTS) is indicated by:

- ❏ A   Wasting of the thenar eminence
- ❏ B   Tinel's sign
- ❏ C   Blanching of all fingers on exposure to cold
- ❏ D   Paraesthesiae of the thumb and index finger
- ❏ E   Pain in the hand, which is worse at night

1.22   With regard to obesity:

- ❏ A   Open surgery is contraindicated
- ❏ B   Laparoscopic surgery is contraindicated
- ❏ C   The risk of morbidity and mortality is decreased
- ❏ D   Weight loss is essential before surgery
- ❏ E   A body mass index (BMI) > 28 is significant

1.23   The following refer to hiatus hernia:

- ❏ A   The treatment of choice is fundoplication
- ❏ B   Rolling hernias are more common than the sliding type
- ❏ C   Severe acid reflux occurs mainly in rolling hernias
- ❏ D   It can be diagnosed by endoscopy
- ❏ E   Weight loss is advised

1.24   Perforated duodenal ulcer:

- ❏ A   May be treated conservatively
- ❏ B   Should be confirmed by gastroscopy before laparotomy
- ❏ C   Should be confirmed by CT before laparotomy
- ❏ D   Can present without abdominal signs
- ❏ E   Is excluded if serum amylase > 500 IU/L

1.25   Ulcerative colitis:

- ❑ A   May be complicated by retinitis
- ❑ B   Should be investigated by rectal biopsy
- ❑ C   May predispose to carcinoma of the large bowel, especially with early onset of total colitis
- ❑ D   Should be investigated by colonoscopy if there is dilatation of the large bowel on plain radiograph
- ❑ E   Is not commonly associated with protein loss

1.26   Common causes of small bowel obstruction in adults are:

- ❑ A   Stricture due to rectal carcinoma
- ❑ B   Adhesions
- ❑ C   Meckel's diverticulum
- ❑ D   Intussusception
- ❑ E   Strangulated hernia

1.27   Recognised consequences of achalasia of the cardia include:

- ❑ A   Dysphagia
- ❑ B   Pneumonia
- ❑ C   Carcinoma of the oesophagus
- ❑ D   Absent gastric air bubble
- ❑ E   Heartburn

1.28   First-degree haemorrhoids are a cause of:

- ❑ A   Rectal bleeding
- ❑ B   Anal pain
- ❑ C   Rectal mucosal prolapse
- ❑ D   Melaena
- ❑ E   Pruritis ani

1.29   Endoscopic retrograde cholangiopancreatography (ERCP):

- ❑ A   Usually requires a general anaesthetic
- ❑ B   Is valuable for confirming a suspicion of acute pancreatitis
- ❑ C   Gives information equivalent to that obtained by percutaneous transhepatic cholangiography
- ❑ D   Is contraindicated in the presence of jaundice
- ❑ E   Can diagnose strictures of the pancreatic duct

1.30   Typical biochemical features of serum in obstructive jaundice include:

- ❏ A   Raised bilirubin
- ❏ B   Increased acid phosphatase
- ❏ C   Increased alkaline phosphatase
- ❏ D   Increased amylase
- ❏ E   Positive hepatitis B surface antigen

1.31   Splenectomy is likely to be of value in:

- ❏ A   Congenital spherocytosis
- ❏ B   Myelofibrosis
- ❏ C   Malaria
- ❏ D   Infectious mononucleosis
- ❏ E   Agranulocytosis

1.32   A lump in the midline of the neck may be:

- ❏ A   A dermoid cyst
- ❏ B   A sebaceous cyst
- ❏ C   A thyroglossal cyst
- ❏ D   A branchial cyst
- ❏ E   A cystic hygroma

1.33   Carcinoma of the breast may present with:

- ❏ A   Peau d'orange
- ❏ B   Shortness of breath
- ❏ C   Lymphoedema of the arm
- ❏ D   A bone fracture
- ❏ E   Inversion of the nipple

1.34   A size 24 Fr catheter:

- ❏ A   Must always be inserted using an aseptic technique
- ❏ B   Is 24 mm in diameter
- ❏ C   Is 24 mm in length
- ❏ D   Is 24 mm in external circumference
- ❏ E   Is the suitable first choice for urethral catheterisation of men

1.35   Renal carcinoma in adults:

- [ ] A   Usually presents as painful haematuria
- [ ] B   Commonly metastasises to bone
- [ ] C   May grow into the inferior vena cava
- [ ] D   May give rise to cannonball metastases
- [ ] E   Is called Wilms' tumour

1.36   A patient has a road traffic accident resulting in severe chest injury. He presents in severe respiratory distress and his trachea is deviated to the left. The first thing that you should do is to:

- [ ] A   Request an urgent radiograph
- [ ] B   Insert an exploratory needle into the second left intercostal space
- [ ] C   Perform an emergency tracheostomy
- [ ] D   Gain intravenous access
- [ ] E   Obtain an ECG

1.37   Varicose veins:

- [ ] A   Cause lipodermatosclerosis
- [ ] B   Should always be treated by injection sclerotherapy
- [ ] C   Are common in rural Africa
- [ ] D   Are more common in the short than in the long saphenous system
- [ ] E   Can cause serious haemorrhage

1.38   Intermittent claudication:

- [ ] A   Is usually caused by atherosclerosis
- [ ] B   Is worse at night
- [ ] C   May improve on continued exercise
- [ ] D   May proceed to gangrene
- [ ] E   Requires surgery to the affected arteries

1.39   Clinical features of acute pancreatitis include:

- [ ] A   Tetany
- [ ] B   Paralytic ileus
- [ ] C   Vomiting
- [ ] D   Jaundice
- [ ] E   A pleural effusion

1.40   Symptoms of malignant change in a melanoma are:

❑   A   Bleeding
❑   B   Hair in the lesion
❑   C   Change in colour
❑   D   Itching
❑   E   Satellite lesions

1.41   A fistula:

❑   A   Arises from a blind-ending abscess cavity
❑   B   Will never heal spontaneously
❑   C   Connects two separate epithelial surfaces
❑   D   May be found in the anal canal
❑   E   May give rise to severe fluid and electrolyte losses

1.42   Physiological or normal saline given intravenously:

❑   A   Is a solution containing 1 mol sodium chloride/L water
❑   B   Is a solution containing 0.9 g sodium chloride/L water
❑   C   Has the same osmotic pressure as plasma
❑   D   Is a 0.9% solution of sodium chloride in water
❑   E   Should never be given for hypovolaemia

1.43   In patients with chronic vomiting:

❑   A   A metabolic acidosis results
❑   B   A metabolic alkalosis results
❑   C   There is excess loss of sodium in the urine
❑   D   Potassium deficiency may occur
❑   E   There may be the same metabolic effect as continual nasogastric aspiration

1.44   Factors that favour wound healing include:

❑   A   A good blood supply
❑   B   A haematoma
❑   C   Tension
❑   D   The presence of bacteria
❑   E   A minimum of suture materials

1.45   Nutritional problems seen after a partial gastrectomy include:

❏ A Macrocytic anaemia
❏ B Osteoporosis
❏ C Weight loss
❏ D Iron deficiency anaemia
❏ E Hypoglycaemia

1.46   The following are features of Horner syndrome on the left side of the face:

❏ A Dilatation of the ipsilateral pupil
❏ B Enophthalmos
❏ C Absent sweating on the affected side of the face
❏ D Deviation of the tongue to one side on protrusion
❏ E Ptosis of the ipsilateral eye

1.47   Tearing of the medial meniscus of the knee leads to:

❏ A Quadriceps wasting
❏ B Recurrent haemarthrosis
❏ C Limitation of knee flexion
❏ D Locking of the knee
❏ E Intermittent effusions

1.48   Neuromuscular blocking agents that act by competitive inhibition include:

❏ A Pethidine
❏ B Suxamethonium
❏ C Neostigmine
❏ D Hexamethonium
❏ E Tubocurarine

1.49   Carcinoma of the stomach is associated with:

❏ A Blood group O
❏ B Cigarette smoking
❏ C Pernicious anaemia
❏ D Iron deficiency anaemia
❏ E Transcoelomic spread to the ovary

13

1.50   Minimally invasive surgery:

☐ A   Is used for cholecystectomy
☐ B   Provides a quicker recovery than an open procedure
☐ C   Can be used for cervical sympathectomy
☐ D   Is contraindicated in morbid obesity
☐ E   Means that minimal skill is required

1.51   A sarcoma:

☐ A   Is a malignant tumour
☐ B   Spreads primarily via the bloodstream
☐ C   Responds to radiotherapy
☐ D   Grows rapidly
☐ E   Has a good prognosis

1.52   Carcinoma of the prostate:

☐ A   Occurs frequently in men aged over 65 years
☐ B   Responds to testosterone therapy
☐ C   Can cause a rectal stricture
☐ D   Produces osteosclerotic secondary bone deposits
☐ E   Spreads to pelvic lymph nodes

1.53   The following classically occur within 24 hours of an operation:

☐ A   Deep vein thrombosis (DVT)
☐ B   Pulmonary embolus (PE)
☐ C   Pulmonary atelectasis
☐ D   Wound dehiscence
☐ E   Reactionary haemorrhage

1.54   Gas gangrene is treated with:

☐ A   Local applications of antiseptics
☐ B   Benzylpenicillin
☐ C   Adequate surgical excision of the wound
☐ D   Primary suture of the wound
☐ E   Blood transfusion

1.55   A benign breast change:

- [ ] A   Often produces cyclical pain
- [ ] B   Is normally unilateral
- [ ] C   Tends to progress in the postmenopausal years
- [ ] D   Is pre-malignant
- [ ] E   Produces diffuse lumpiness

1.56   An abdominal aortic aneurysm:

- [ ] A   May be seen on a plain abdominal radiograph
- [ ] B   May present with a collapsing pulse
- [ ] C   May be the result of syphilis
- [ ] D   Needs treatment only if it causes back pain
- [ ] E   Usually involves the renal arteries

1.57   A nasogastric tube:

- [ ] A   Should be used to protect respiratory function in all patients with severe head injury
- [ ] B   Should be spigotted and aspirated at regular intervals
- [ ] C   May be used for feeding
- [ ] D   Is required in upper gastrointestinal bleeding to assess blood loss
- [ ] E   May be used in the treatment of large bowel obstruction

1.58   The following facts are true of pleomorphic adenomas and their treatment:

- [ ] A   They occur in the parotid gland
- [ ] B   They grow rapidly
- [ ] C   They can be safely removed by simple enucleation
- [ ] D   Surgery may result in damage to the facial nerve
- [ ] E   Surgery may result in Frey syndrome

1.59   Carcinoma of the oesophagus:

- [ ] A   Occurs most frequently in the middle third of the oesophagus
- [ ] B   Is predominantly squamous in type
- [ ] C   Is a complication of oesophagitis
- [ ] D   Is associated with alcohol intake
- [ ] E   Occurs in Plummer–Vinson syndrome

1.60   In acute cholecystitis:

❏ A   Immediate cholecystectomy may be performed
❏ B   Antibiotics are mandatory
❏ C   Delayed cholecystectomy may be performed
❏ D   Treatment includes laparoscopic cholecystectomy
❏ E   Laparotomy is advisable

————————————— **END** —————————————

**Go over your answers until your time is up. Correct answers
and teaching notes are overleaf.**

BEST OF FIVE AND MULTIPLE CHOICE QUESTIONS PAPER 1
Answers

The correct answer options for each question are given below.

1.1	E		1.31	A B
1.2	E		1.32	A B C
1.3	A		1.33	A B C D E
1.4	A		1.34	A
1.5	D		1.35	B C D
1.6	B		1.36	None correct
1.7	C		1.37	A E
1.8	D		1.38	A C D
1.9	C		1.39	A B C D E
1.10	B		1.40	A C D E
1.11	E		1.41	C D E
1.12	D		1.42	C D
1.13	D		1.43	B D E
1.14	E		1.44	A E
1.15	C		1.45	A C D E
1.16	C		1.46	B C E
1.17	A C D E		1.47	A B C D E
1.18	C D E		1.48	E
1.19	A B E		1.49	B C D E
1.20	A B D E		1.50	A B C
1.21	A B D E		1.51	A B C D
1.22	E		1.52	A C D E
1.23	D E		1.53	C E
1.24	A D		1.54	B C
1.25	B C		1.55	A E
1.26	B E		1.56	A C
1.27	A B C D E		1.57	C E
1.28	A E		1.58	A D E
1.29	E		1.59	A B D E
1.30	A C		1.60	A B C D

BEST OF FIVE AND MULTIPLE CHOICE QUESTIONS PAPER 1
Answers and Teaching Notes

1.1   E: Rupturing abdominal aortic aneurysm

Abdominal aortic aneurysms have a high incidence of rupture once they reach or exceed 6 cm. Often the first manifestation is excruciating back pain, as the blood leaks into the retroperitoneal space before the aneurysm blows out into the peritoneal cavity. The combination of a big aneurysm and sudden severe back pain should always lead to this diagnosis.

Acute cholecystitis is just a distractor because the patient has already had cholecystectomy. Acute pancreatitis is a less likely diagnosis because the patient does not have risk factors for acute pancreatitis. The pain from a herniated lumbar disc usually runs down the leg and is exacerbated by coughing or sneezing. The pain of acute appendicitis is usually felt in the right iliac fossa.

1.2   E: Taeniae coli

The taeniae coli are three bands of longitudinal muscle on the surface of the large intestine. The large intestine does not have a continuous layer of longitudinal muscle – instead, it has taeniae coli. These three bands meet at the appendix, which projects from the dependent portion of the caecum.

The omental appendages are fatty appendages that are unique to the large intestine. These are all over the large intestine and not specifically associated with the appendix. The haustra are multiple pouches in the wall of the large intestine, which form where the longitudinal muscle layer of the wall of the large intestine is deficient. Remember, the taeniae coli, omental appendages and haustra are the three distinctive features of the large intestine!

The ileal orifice is the space where the ileum open into the caecum – it is surrounded by the ileocecal valve. The semilunar folds are the folds found along the lining of the large intestine.

1.3 A: Extracorporeal shock wave lithotripsy

Extracoproreal shock wave lithotripsy is the most commonly used technique for fragmenting urinary stones and allowing their passage. Pregnancy and coagulopathy are contraindications for this technique, which are absent in this patient.

Retrograde endoscopic approaches are more invasive than extracorporeal shock wave lithotripsy. Open removal would have been a good option for a much larger stone. Waiting for spontaneous passage would have been a perfect option for a much smaller stone (3 mm). An 8 mm stone way up at the pelviureteric junction has a very small chance of spontaneous passage.

1.4 A: Median nerve

Carpal tunnel syndrome is caused by compression of the median nerve within the carpal tunnel, which is a canal on the anterior side of the wrist. It is made of the carpal bones, which are covered by the flexor retinaculum. It contains the tendon of flexor pollicis longus, the tendons of flexor digitorum superficialis and profundus, and the median nerve. If the sheath over the common flexor tendons, the ulnar bursa, becomes inflamed, this can compress the median nerve in the canal, leading to pain and weakness in the hand. None of the other structures mentioned in the question is contained in the carpal tunnel, so they would not be compressed in that space.

1.5 D: Placement of nasogastric tube

The most likely aetiology is postoperative adhesions that have caused obstruction. Placement of a nasogastric tube (NGT) to decompress the bowel will be the next most appropriate step in management, and in most patients this will lead to gradual and complete resolution of the bowel obstruction.

Surgical exploration is indicated if there is clinical deterioration after the placement of the NGT. Surgery should not be undertaken until a trial of conservative therapy with small bowel decompression and a period of nil by mouth have been attempted. The investigations, abdominal CT, barium enema and small bowel series, are helpful but must be performed after the placement of the NGT.

1.6 B: Pulmonary embolism

Immobilisation after fracture, particularly in elderly people, is a significant risk for development of DVT, followed by PE.

Signs and symptoms of an infectious disease were not present and therefore TB is a less likely possibility. Elderly people are at risk of pneumonia when in hospital, but the course is marked by signs and symptoms of an infection, which were absent in this woman. Congestive heart failure is a possibility in elderly people, but in the setting given is unlikely to be the cause of the sudden death. Older people are at risk of cancer, but this course suggests immobilisation leading to pulmonary thromboembolism.

1.7   C: Chronic bacterial prostatitis

Chronic bacterial prostatitis should be considered in men who have a history of recurrent bacteriuria. A chronically infected prostate can serve as the source of pathogens for recurrent urinary tract infections (UTIs). A pattern of relapsing UTIs in a middle-aged man strongly suggests chronic bacterial prostatitis. *E. coli* is a typical organism associated with UTIs. The PSA can be slightly elevated with prostatic inflammation.

Prostatic hyperplasia can produce an enlarged prostate, but it is usually non-tender. The obstruction caused by an enlarged prostate can predispose to recurrent UTIs. The PSA can be slightly elevated with nodular hyperplasia, and is typically elevated to more than twice the normal value when prostatic adenocarcinoma is present. The presence of a palpable nodule suggests a carcinoma. Prostatic adenocarcinomas are usually non-tender. Patients who have signs and symptoms of prostatitis but no evidence of prostatic inflammation (normal leukocyte counts) and negative urine cultures, are classified as having prostodynia. A urothelial carcinoma of the urethra is uncommon. Haematuria is often present and may cause obstruction and predispose to UTIs.

1.8   D: Ionised calcium

The parathyroids can be inadvertently removed or traumatised with thyroid surgery, resulting in hypocalcaemia. Post-surgical monitoring of calcium levels is routinely performed.

Calcitonin is not involved in acute symptoms of decreased serum calcium. The TSH will not be acutely altered and will stabilise with thyroid replacement therapy. Changes in thyroxine levels do not explain these acute findings. The parathyroid hormone may be decreased eventually, but measurement is of no value acutely.

1.9   C: Hypospadias

Hypospadias is a malformation that affects the urethral tube and the foreskin on a male's penis. It is a disorder in which the male urethral opening is not located at the tip of the penis; instead it can be located anywhere along the urethra. Most commonly with hypospadias, the opening is located along the underside of the penis, near the tip. Hypospadias is a disorder that primarily affects newborn boys. It occurs in about 1 in every 150–300 boys. Hypospadias also has a genetic component. Eight per cent of fathers of boys with hypospadias also had the condition. Some studies show an increased risk for siblings to be born with hypospadias after the birth of one child with the problem.

Some newborn boys who have other congenital abnormalities such as undescended testes or inguinal hernias may also have hypospadias. Infection is a common complication, and partial urethral stricture may lead to urinary tract obstruction.

Exstrophy is opening of the bladder through a defect in the lower abdominal wall. Phimosis may be an anomaly, but it is more commonly the result of inflammation with scarring in uncircumcised males. Epispadias is defined as an abnormal opening of the urethra on to the dorsal aspect of the penis. Cryptorchidism is failure of normal descent of the testes into the scrotal sac. It occurs in about 1 in 200 males.

1.10 B: Perforation of a colonic diverticulum

The history of chronic constipation points to the presence of diverticular disease of the colon. The clinical picture suggests perforation of a colonic diverticulum, as indicated by free gas under the diaphragm on the abdominal radiograph.

Crohn's disease is more often diagnosed in people between the ages of 20 and 30. The most common symptoms of Crohn's disease are abdominal pain, often in the lower right area, and diarrhoea. Rectal bleeding, weight loss, arthritis, skin problems and fever may also occur. Bleeding may be serious and persistent, leading to anaemia. Hirschsprung's disease or congenital megacolon is caused by the absence of nerve cells (called ganglia cells) in the large intestine, which stimulate the rhythmic contraction that moves material through the gut (peristalsis). These ganglia cells may be absent from either just a short segment of large intestine or all of it. Hirschsprung's disease causes a quarter of all cases of newborn intestinal obstruction, although the condition may not be detected until later in infancy or childhood. It occurs five times more frequently in boys than in girls. Appendicitis will cause pain in the right lower quadrant. There is no association between pancreatitis and the symptoms described in this patient. Pancreatitis usually presents with upper abdominal pain that often radiates to the back.

1.11 E: Ventilation–perfusion scan

This patient most probably had a PE. The risk factors for PE in this patient are obesity and surgery. Clinical features are highly suggestive of the diagnosis. The most appropriate diagnostic test will be a ventilation–perfusion scan to confirm clinical suspicion.

A chest radiograph will show an area of infarction secondary to a PE as a wedge-shaped defect. However, in most instances the chest radiograph is normal and non-specific. A CT scan, similar to a chest radiograph, may show an area of infarction but is not the most appropriate diagnostic test in this scenario. An ECG strip will show tachycardia and possible right axis deviation caused by pulmonary hypertension, and right ventricular strain with ST–T wave changes. However, it is not diagnostic. MRI is not the test of choice to diagnose PE.

1.12 D: Insertion of a chest drain

The patient, although haemodynamically stable, needs contaminated blood as well as air in the pleural space to be drained. If contaminated blood is left in the pleural space, it can have devastating consequences as a result of the development of empyema. A chest drain inserted appropriately will drain the blood and air. Furthermore, drainage from the chest drain can guide the treating physician with regard to further aggressive therapy such as exploratory thoracotomy if bleeding is persistent or massive in volume (1000–1500 mL). Almost 85–90% of stab wounds to the chest can be managed with just the insertion of a chest drain.

The patient is breathing spontaneously with acceptable saturations on room air and, therefore, mechanical ventilation is out of the question. Antibiotics will have to be prescribed but only after the blood and air have been drained from the pleural space.

1.13 D: Colonoscopy

Iron deficiency anaemia in a man is always the result of chronic blood loss, and in this patient the source is the gastrointestinal tract. The presence of altered bowel habits and the absence of other symptoms suggest a colonic pathology, most probably a cancer, which will be best seen by colonoscopy. Upper gastrointestinal endoscopy, barium swallow and abdominal radiograph will be normal in his case. Abdominal angiography is an expensive and invasive test that is usually indicated to identify a source of bleeding in patients with massive blood loss (> 2 mL/min).

1.14 E: Peptic oesophageal stricture

The history of this patient suggests peptic oesophageal stricture. This benign stricture develops in patients with acid peptic disease and is best treated with endoscopic dilatation of the stricture and aggressive treatment of gastro-oesophageal reflux disease.

Diffuse oesophageal spasm will produce dysphagia for both solids and liquids, and is usually accompanied by squeezing chest pain. Oesophageal squamous carcinoma is less likely to be the cause as the patient is young and does not smoke. A lower oesophageal web will produce episodic dysphagia because foods that are larger in size than the diameter of the web will become lodged in the distal oesophagus. Scleroderma is three times more common in women than in men and will be accompanied by Raynaud's phenomenon and characteristic skin changes.

1.15 C: Injury to major bronchus

The presentation is suggestive of injury to a major bronchus. This type of injury is seen when a major blow to the chest occurs at a time when the glottis is closed. If not recognised initially because of the presence of surgical emphysema, such an injury becomes evident once the air leak persists or gets worse on connecting the drain to suction when the lung fails to expand.

Air embolism is less likely in this patient and massive air embolism is usually lethal. Oesophageal injury will result in surgical emphysema but not major air leak. Fat embolism is a possibility in multiple trauma victims; however, the presentation will include respiratory failure, cerebral dysfunction and petechiae. None of these is present in this patient. A tension pneumothorax occurs secondary to blunt or penetrating injury of the lung, which results in a one-way valve being created. Air leaks from the lung into the pleural space and is unable to escape, resulting in increased intrapleural pressure. Intrapleural pressure eventually increases to the point where it interferes with venous return, resulting in blood pooling in capacitance vessels and ensuing cardiovascular collapse and shock.

1.16 Management of a patient with a head injury   Answer: C

In the patient with a head injury, trauma management follows the standard ABC protocol: A (airway), B (breathing), C (circulation). It is important to immobilise the neck during resuscitation. The response to hypovolaemia is tachycardia and hypotension, which is graded according to severity as follows:

	I < 15%	II 15–30%	III 30–40%	IV > 40%
Heart rate (beats/min)	< 100	Raised > 100	Raised > 120	Raised > 140
Blood pressure	Normal	Normal/Low	Low	Low
Respiratory rate (/min)	Normal	Normal/Raised	Raised 30–40	Raised > 40
Peripheral circulation	Normal	Cool, pale	Cool, pale	Cold, clammy 'SHOCK'

Hypertension and bradycardia suggest raised intracranial pressure. Pain can cause raised blood pressure and tachycardia, but careful neurological examination is necessary.

The GCS score is calculated as follows:

Eye response:
1 No response
2 Open to pain
3 Open to command
4 Open spontaneously

Verbal:
1 No sounds
2 Incomprehensible sounds
3 Inappropriate words
4 Confused conversation
5 Oriented conversation

Motor response:
1 No response
2 Extension to pain (decerebrate)
3 Abnormal flexion to pain (decorticate)
4 Flexion withdrawal response to pain
5 Localises pain
6 Obeys commands

Investigations depend on the history and clinical examination findings. Loss of consciousness and retrograde amnesia suggest increased severity of injury. Neurological signs warrant CT.

Exposure is necessary to make an accurate assessment of injury. A helmet should be removed, paying particular attention to neck immobilisation.

1.17 Acute appendicitis   Answers: A C D E

Pain often starts vaguely in the central abdomen (as the appendix is a midgut structure) and then localises to the right iliac fossa (RIF), when the peritoneum becomes inflamed.

The absence of some of the typical symptoms and signs does not exclude a diagnosis of appendicitis. Symptoms include:

- RIF pain
- nausea and vomiting
- loss of appetite
- diarrhoea may occur.

Signs include:

- tachycardia
- flushed peripheries (especially the face)
- pyrexia – usually up to 37.5°C
- fetor oris
- mildly raised WCC.

The differential diagnosis for RIF pain is ovulation/ovarian cyst rupture or pelvic inflammatory disease. This is often difficult to differentiate and may require further investigations such as ultrasonography or CT to assist in making the diagnosis.

In cases where the diagnosis is in doubt, laparoscopy is particularly useful, proceeding to the definitive procedure. Laparoscopic appendicectomy is increasingly used.

In young children, an upper respiratory tract infection may cause mesenteric adenitis, which presents with pain in the RIF and can be easily mistaken for appendicitis. Other similar conditions are Meckel's diverticulitis, Crohn's ileitis and gastroenteritis.

1.18 Chest drain   Answers: C D E

The treatment of pneumothorax includes the following:

- Aspiration – in uncomplicated cases with < 20% pneumothorax, this may suffice
- Intercostal tube drainage
- Pleurodesis – used in persistent recurrent cases.

A chest drain is inserted using local anaesthetic. General anaesthetic is not essential. A small incision is made just above the rib. Blunt dissection is performed though the intercostal muscles and parietal pleura, using artery forceps. The end of the chest drain is then guided into the chest. The drain should be attached to an underwater seal and secured in position. A chest radiograph is performed to confirm the position. The movement of fluid in the drainage tube on breathing and bubbles in the drainage bottle suggest correct placement.

It is essential to insert a chest drain **after** emergency relief of tension pneumothorax. Tension pneumothorax is treated with immediate insertion of a cannula in the second intercostal space in the mid-clavicular line. After release of the air under tension, a formal chest drain must be inserted.

Empyema is pus found within the pleural cavity. It can be treated by 'closed tube drainage' or percutaneous drainage inserted under radiological control.

Chest injuries may be associated with a pneumothorax or haemothorax (or both).

1.19 Clinical features of hyperthyroidism   Answers: A B E

The clinical features of thyroid disease are determined by examination of the thyroid gland itself and examination of all the systems for signs of altered thyroid status.

The thyroid gland itself may be normal or enlarged, with a single nodule or a multinodular goitre. It may have a bruit.

Hyperthyroidism causes:

- nervousness/anxiety/tremor
- increased appetite
- weight loss
- preference for cold weather
- palpitations.

Eye signs are:

- exophthalmos (Graves' disease)
- lid retraction
- lid lag
- dilated pupils
- ophthalmoplegia.

Hand signs are:

- tremor
- sweating
- acropachy (clubbing of fingers)
- onycholysis.

Cardiovascular system signs are:

- tachycardia
- rapid sleeping pulse rate

- heart failure
- atrial fibrillation.

1.20 Clinical features of prolapsed intervertebral disc at the L5–S1 level   Answers: A B D E

Acute prolapse of the intervertebral disc causes severe back pain, with pain in the buttock and the back of the leg – sciatica. The clinical features are:

- muscle weakness and wasting
- reduced ankle reflex
- sensory loss on the outer leg and dorsum of the foot.

Herniation at L4–5 will compress the fifth lumbar nerve root and at L5–S1 the first sacral root. Straight-leg raising is painful.

L5 signs: weakness of ankle dorsiflexion and big toe extension; increased knee jerk as a result of weak antagonists; and sensory loss on the outer leg and medial part of the foot.

S1 signs: weakness of plantar flexion and weakness of inversion of the foot; depressed ankle jerk; and sensory loss on the lateral border of the foot.

Cauda equina compression causes urinary retention and sensory loss near the sacrum.

Acute disc prolapse may cause paravetebral muscle spasm. Straight-leg raising causes pain and is restricted and may produce paraplegia.

Investigations include:

- radiograph
- CT
- MRI
- myelography.

Treatment includes:

- heat
- analgesia
- exercises
- rest
- reduction (bed rest and traction)
- removal of the disc prolapse by laminectomy or discectomy.

The patient will require rehabilitation.

1.21 Carpal tunnel syndrome

Answers: A B D E

In CTS the median nerve, which passes deep to the flexor retinaculum, is compressed.

Causes of CTS are:

- idiopathic
- pregnancy
- rheumatoid arthritis
- amyloid
- collagen disorders
- hypothyroidism
- oedema.

In the hand, the median nerve supplies the muscles of the radial two lumbricals. It also carries sympathetic nerve fibres to the hand and supplies flexor muscles of the forearm (except flexor carpi ulnaris and the ulnar half of flexor digitorum profundus). The following are features of CTS:

- Wasting of the thenar eminence
- Pain in the hand, which is classically worse at night, associated with burning and tingling
- Loss of blanching of the lateral fingers on exposure to cold
- Tinel's sign – this consists of tingling in the hand produced by continuous tapping over the flexor retinaculum
- Paraesthesiae/numbness in the thumb and lateral two and a half fingers
- Weakness of thumb abduction.

The median nerve roots are C6, C7, C8 and T1. The nerve passes lateral to the brachial artery in the upper arm and then crosses superficially at the mid-humerus level to lie on the medial aspect of the brachial artery.

1.22 Obesity

Answer: E:

Obesity is becoming significantly more common in the general population. The treatment of choice is conservative, encouraging weight loss, diet improvement and exercise programmes. However, surgical treatment may be necessary and presents its own problems and complications. As always, these should be considered as 'early' and 'late' as well as 'general' and 'specific'. The complications are as follows:

- Operative:
    - general anaesthesia, eg difficulty with intubation, requiring 'rapid sequence induction', and difficult cannulation

- drug metabolism is altered, requiring higher doses and intravenous access
- surgery – technically difficult as a result of obscured access; takes longer.
- Postoperative:
  - DVT and PE risk is increased, especially as a result of slow mobilisation
  - wound infection
  - wound dehiscence
  - haematoma formation
- Medical: there is a predisposition to:
  - cardiac disease, eg hypertension, ischaemic heart disease
  - respiratory disease – as a result of inadequate respiratory effort
  - diabetes
  - gallstones.

Surgery may be required to treat obesity (eg gastric stapling) or may be essential in obese patients who present in the emergency situation (eg strangulated hernia). Laparoscopic surgery can be performed in obese patients and this may be advantageous, but it requires skill and special long instruments for adequate access.

In elective cases, weight loss should be encouraged with the help of a dietitian and a weight loss programme. A BMI > 28 increases the risks of surgery. Gross obesity doubles the risk of morbidity and mortality.

1.23 Hiatus hernia   **Answers: D E**

Hiatus hernia is classified into two types:

1. Sliding: 90% are of this type. The gastro-oesophageal junction (GOJ) slides upwards into the thorax, rendering it incompetent, resulting in acid reflux and its complications (see Question 4.35, Paper 4). Management of any surgical case involves conservative measures first, then medical treatment and surgical intervention:
   - conservative measures include weight reduction (to decrease the intra-abdominal pressure) and raising the head of the bed
   - medical treatment includes drugs such as H_2-receptor antagonists or proton pump inhibitors to counteract acid reflux
   - surgical treatment is Nissen's fundoplication. There are variations on this procedure but essentially the GOJ is pulled back into the abdomen and the fundus of the stomach is wrapped around it. This can be done by open surgery, but is increasingly carried out laparoscopically.

2. Rolling (paraoesophageal): 10% are of this type; more common in obese women. The fundus of the stomach rotates in front of the oesophagus and herniates through the oesophageal hiatus up into the mediastinum. Note that the oesophageal sphincter is not affected and so reflux is not usually a problem. This type of hernia can be asymptomatic but occasionally the stomach can strangulate.

1.24 Perforated duodenal ulcer   Answers: A D

Perforation is an important complication of duodenal ulceration. It may present without abdominal signs, particularly in elderly people and those on steroids. However, patients often present with peritonitis, the features of which are severe constant pain, rebound tenderness, guarding and rigidity, and absent bowel sounds. Other important features are tachycardia, hypotension and pyrexia. Abnormal investigations include leukocytosis, raised amylase (not as high as in pancreatitis), abnormal features on chest radiograph (gas under the diaphragm in 90%) and signs of free air on the abdominal radiograph (bowel gas shadows). Gastroscopy is indicated for bleeding ulcers, not perforation.

Management may be conservative, eg in elderly people or those unfit for surgery, symptomatic relief is provided while healing occurs as the omentum seals off the perforation. Surgery involves laparotomy with simple oversewing of the perforation.

1.25 Ulcerative colitis   Answers: B C

Ulcerative colitis is an inflammatory disease of the mucosa and submucosa of the large bowel. It is often complicated by systemic features, including anaemia (of chronic disease or of iron deficiency due to rectal bleeding), seronegative arthropathy (20%), uveitis and iritis, skin lesions (eg erythema nodosum and pyoderma gangrenosum) and, occasionally, sclerosing cholangitis.

Specific investigations include:

- Full blood count (FBC) for anaemia, urea and electrolytes (U&Es), erythrocyte sedimentation rate (ESR) as a measure of disease activity, rectal examination followed by proctoscopy and sigmoidoscopy with a biopsy if necessary
- Abdominal radiograph may show colonic dilatation of toxic megacolon
- Stool culture to exclude an infective cause

- Contrast study: an urgent barium enema may be performed without bowel preparation, ie an 'instant enema', only if there is no toxic dilatation on a plain film. This may show loss of haustra, a lead-pipe colon or filling defects resulting from pseudopolyps or carcinoma
- Flexible colonoscopy: this is very useful to visualise bowel and permits excision of lesions such as polyps; it is used for surveillance. However, it carries the risk of perforation in fulminant cases of ulcerative colitis.

In young patients who have had total colitis for 10 years, the risk of developing carcinoma of the colon or rectum is about 10%.

Protein loss occurs as bowel mucosa is disrupted and sloughs off with blood.

1.26 Small bowel obstruction   Answers: B E

Please read the question carefully. It is advisable to know a list of causes but beware of the question that has been altered slightly. The answers can often be worked out logically. In 'A' the question refers to the small bowel and rectal carcinoma occurs in the large bowel!

Adhesions are a common cause of bowel obstruction. Meckel's diverticulum is associated with a congenital band, which may cause small bowel obstruction but this is not common (the most common complication of Meckel's diverticulum is inflammation).

Intussusception is when a segment of bowel becomes invaginated into the bowel distal to it, ie 'telescoping'. This answer is false because it is not common in adults, but it does commonly occur in children.

1.27 Achalasia   Answers: A B C D E

Achalasia is a disorder of oesophageal motility, resulting in contraction of the lower oesophageal sphincter. The proximal section becomes dilated. Patients are unable to tolerate either solids or fluids so that dysphagia is usually the presenting symptom. Fluids may spill over into the trachea, causing aspiration pneumonia. Vomiting and retrosternal pain may occur in severe cases. A chest radiograph will show a widened mediastinum and possibly a fluid level in the oesophagus. A barium swallow shows a 'beak' appearance with dilatation of the oesophagus and a tapering constriction. The constriction prevents the passage of air into the stomach. There is an association between achalasia and oesophageal carcinoma.

1.28 First-degree haemorrhoids   Answers: A E

Haemorrhoids (piles) are abnormal dilated cushions of veins at the lower end of the anal mucosal columns. Symptoms of haemorrhoids include perianal irritation and itching (pruritus ani), pain, prolapse and bleeding. They are classified according to their position:

- First-degree haemorrhoids are not visible; they bleed after defecation and do not cause pain
- Second-degree haemorrhoids prolapse after defecation, but then reduce spontaneously
- Third-degree haemorrhoids prolapse and remain external
- Fourth-degree haemorrhoids thrombose after prolapse.

Option 'C' is false by definition. Haemorrhoids are usually located at the 3, 7 and 11 o'clock positions. They are situated above the dentate line and so can be injected painlessly. Pain occurs when they thrombose.

The following are management options:

- Conservative: high-fibre diet, avoidance of straining and good anal hygiene
- Medical: local anaesthetic agents, steroids and symptomatic relief
- Surgical: submucosal injection or banding is used for first- and second-degree haemorrhoids; haemorrhoidectomy is used for third- and fourth-degree haemorrhoids.

1.29 Endoscopic retrograde cholangiopancreatography   Answer: E

The investigation of the biliary tree includes:

- Abdominal radiograph: only 10% of gallstones are radio-opaque
- Ultrasonography: very useful to make the diagnosis of gallstones
- ERCP: used for imaging of the biliary tree and pancreatic ducts. It involves injection of contrast to outline the ducts. It allows the ampullary region of the pancreas to be inspected visually and the pancreatic duct may be outlined. It is helpful for identifying stones, strictures and tumours that cause obstruction, as well as for therapeutic intervention, eg stone extraction or stent insertion where there is a blockage. Endoscopic sphincterotomy can be performed. It is particularly useful in the jaundiced patient and in those patients who are unfit for surgery
- Percutaneous transhepatic cholangiography (PTC): often used where ERCP fails, but it is more invasive. It involves entry via the skin into the liver and then injection of contrast into the duct system. There is no

visual information about the pancreas. Stents can be placed via PTC but sphincterotomy cannot be performed
- Cholangiography: this can be done operatively or via a T tube.

1.30 Obstructive jaundice   Answers: A C

In obstructive jaundice there is obstruction to bile drainage, preventing its normal flow into the duodenum. This is also known as 'extrahepatic' jaundice. As expected there is a rise in serum bilirubin, which is of the conjugated type as liver function is maintained. The urine appears dark because the excessive bilirubin is excreted by the kidney. The faeces are pale as a result of the lack of stercobilin, which causes the brown coloration. (Note that urobilinogen is increased in the urine in liver cell damage and haemolytic anaemia. It is initially colourless in urine but darkens on standing.)

In obstructive jaundice, liver function tests must be performed. Typically they show:

- Bilirubin: raised
- Alkaline phosphatase: raised (liver isoenzyme)
- Transaminases: mild-to-moderate rise.

Acid phosphatase is raised in prostatic carcinoma. Amylase is a pancreatic enzyme that may or may not be raised in obstructive jaundice, depending on the cause of the obstruction. It is by no means typical. Hepatitis B causes infective hepatitis, resulting in liver damage and intrahepatic jaundice.

1.31 Spleen   Answers: A B

The spleen is a specialised lymphoid organ. It is highly vascular and is required for the maturation of white blood cells and for the destruction of effete red blood cells. Splenectomy is indicated for the following:

- Hypersplenism/splenomegaly
- Staging of lymphoma
- Excision of tumours, cysts or abscesses.

Splenectomy may be useful in the following conditions:

- Congenital spherocytosis
- Autoimmune thrombocytosis
- Autoimmune haemolysis
- Portal hypertension
- Splenic vein hypertension

- Gaucher's disease
- Myelofibrosis
- Trauma.

Splenic rupture is an indication for splenectomy. This may be a result of rib injuries, blunt trauma or perioperative injury. Certain infections, such as Epstein–Barr virus (EBV), malaria and infectious mononucleosis render the spleen susceptible to spontaneous rupture, but splenectomy will not alter the underlying disease as the question implies.

In agranulocytosis, white blood cells are deficient and hence splenectomy would be detrimental.

1.32 Neck lump   Answers: A B C

Dermoid cysts may arise from epithelium along lines of embryological development. They may arise in the midline of the head and neck and may contain hair or other ectodermal structures.

Sebaceous cysts are the most common skin cysts; they consist of stratified squamous lining epithelium filled with keratin. They are covered by normal epithelium and often have a punctum. They can occur anywhere but tend to occur where hair follicles are present.

A thyroglossal cyst occurs in the midline. It is situated anywhere along the midline, usually beneath the hyoid bone along the thyroglossal tract. This is the embryological tract of descent of the thyroid gland from the foramen caecum to its position in the neck. A diagnostic feature is that it moves on swallowing or protrusion of the tongue.

A branchial cyst arises from the remnants of the second pharyngeal pouch. It is typically a painless soft swelling, appearing deep to the sternomastoid muscle and bulging forward at the anterior border.

Cystic hygromas are lymphangiomas. They are present at birth and may be huge. They occur below the angle of the mandible on the side of the neck and not in the midline.

1.33 Carcinoma of the breast   Answers: A B C D E

Carcinoma of the breast may present with local symptoms, eg a lump, nipple discharge/inversion or skin changes, or metastatic symptoms such as shortness of breath.

Paget's disease produces an eczematous change around the nipple. Locally advanced tumours may cause skin ulceration or even necrosis.

Axillary or supraclavicular lymphadenopathy may be presenting features. Lymphoedema of the arm may be caused by the following:

- Surgery for breast cancer
- Radiotherapy to the axilla for breast cancer
- Axillary node disease.

Distant spread most commonly occurs to the:

- bone (sclerotic as well as lytic lesions)
- liver
- lungs (discrete metastases or lymphangitis)
- brain.

Bone metastases may cause fractures as a presenting symptom.

1.34 Urinary catheters   Answer: A

A urinary catheter must always be inserted using an aseptic technique to prevent the introduction of infection. Usually a size 14 F or 16 French catheter is appropriate for catheterisation of the male urethra. The French size (divided by 3) indicates the diameter in millimetres.

Advice should be sought if there has been recent prostate surgery, there is a urethral stricture or the patient has a history of difficult catheterisation, when suprapubic catheterisation would be more appropriate.

1.35 Renal carcinoma   Answers: B C D

Renal carcinoma is more common in men than in women; the incidence increases after the age of 40. It is an adenocarcinoma, also known as a hypernephroma because of its resemblance, under the microscope, to adrenal tissue.

Presenting features include the following:

- Haematuria, which is usually painless and may be macroscopic or microscopic
- Loin pain
- Abdominal mass
- Pyrexia of unknown origin
- Hypertension resulting from excess renin
- Polycythaemia resulting from excess erythropoietin
- Hypercalcaemia
- Secondaries, eg cannonball metastases in the lung seen on a chest radiograph or bone metastases

- A left-sided varicocele; this is because the left testicular vein drains into the left renal vein, whereas the right testicular vein drains directly into the inferior vena cava (IVC); an obstruction to venous drainage by a left-sided tumour will cause back pressure and hence varicosities of the left testicular vein, producing a left-sided varicocele. Both renal veins drain into the IVC.

1.36 Chest injury   Answer: None correct

In any case of trauma the primary survey consists of assessment of:

A   airway
B   breathing
C   circulation.

The first action is to check the airway and then to ensure breathing. Often these are checked simultaneously. Answers 'B' and 'D' are essential but not the first procedure. If tension pneumothorax is suspected, insertion of a cannula is a matter of urgency. Intravenous access is often already established by paramedics.

It is important to remember protection of the cervical spine. The patient must be resuscitated to achieve stability of all the above. After this, a secondary survey must be carried out to assess the patient from head to toe. This may be tailored to more specific areas suggested by the history and examination. The presenting features of a tension pneumothorax are severe shortness of breath and shock. The classic signs of a right-sided pneumothorax include decreased chest wall movement, tracheal deviation to the left and hyper-resonance on the right, with absent breath sounds. This is an emergency and requires immediate insertion of a cannula into the second intercostal space on the affected side. After this, a chest radiograph may be obtained.

Note that you should not request a chest radiograph to diagnose a tension pneumothorax!

1.37 Varicose veins   Answers: A E

Varicose veins are dilated superficial veins of the legs. They result from incompetence of the valves between the superficial and deep systems of venous drainage. The long saphenous system is involved in 90% of cases and the short saphenous system in 10%. Previous DVT predisposes to superficial vein congestion.

Varicose veins are a disease of developed countries. Injection sclerotherapy is of use only in minor varicose veins.

Complications include pain (dull ache), cramps, ankle oedema, haemorrhage, thrombophlebitis, lipodermatosclerosis and ulceration.

1.38 Intermittent claudication   Answers: A C D

Intermittent claudication is characteristically described as pain in the lower limbs that occurs on exercise and is relieved by rest. The pain often occurs in the calf, but can also occur in the thigh or buttock. It is caused by atherosclerosis. The outcome varies:

- A third undergo spontaneous remission.
- A third can tolerate the symptoms.
- A third experience significant disability and restriction in their daily lives.

These patients go on to develop 'rest pain' and often hang their feet over the side of the bed to ease the pain (increasing the blood flow). If left untreated, they may develop necrosis or gangrene and require amputation. Some patients are able to 'walk through their pain'. This encourages the formation of collateral circulation and may help the symptoms.

1.39 Pancreatitis   Answers: A B C D E

Acute pancreatitis presents as an acute abdomen, with pain in the epigastrium or upper abdomen radiating to the back. It is worsened by movement, and the patient can find no relief.

Vomiting is common.

Paralytic ileus is fairly common and bowel sounds are absent or diminished.

Activated pancreatic enzymes are released into the pancreas, causing inflammation.

Hypocalcaemia develops if there is extensive fat necrosis because calcium is then sequestered. This may result in tetany. The complications of pancreatitis are:

- pseudocyst formation
- intra-abdominal bleeding
- acute respiratory distress syndrome (ARDS)
- renal failure.

Inflammation of the pancreas with oedema (or a mass in the head of the pancreas) may result in obstruction to the flow of bile and thus cause jaundice.

1.40 Malignant melanoma — Answers: A C D E

A change in the characteristics of a mole may be an indication of malignancy.

Changes include the following:

- Surface characteristics, eg increase in size, shape or thickness
- Change in colour (eg darkening in patches) or pigmentation
- Itching
- Bleeding
- Brown halo appearance around the lesion
- Satellite lesions – these are caused by lateral spread around the lesion.

1.41 Fistula — Answers: C D E

A fistula is an abnormal connection between two epithelial surfaces. It is lined with granulation tissue and can become epithelialised. A fistula persists if the contents continue to flow along the tract, ie if there is distal obstruction to the normal outflow of the contents. If a fistula occurs between two loops of bowel (eg small bowel and colon) large amounts of fluid may be lost. A fistula in the anal canal is also known as a 'fistula *in ano*'. It connects the lumen of the anal canal with skin. Anal fistulae are classified into two main groups:

1. **Low**: below the anorectal ring; this type is amenable to surgery by 'laying open' the fistula, which then heals by secondary intention.
2. **High**: above the anorectal ring; this is extremely difficult to treat because surgery may render the patient incontinent.

In contrast, a sinus is a blind-ending tract that connects a cavity with an epithelial surface.

1.42 Normal or physiological saline — Answers: C D

Normal or physiological saline is a solution containing 0.9% NaCl in water. This means that there is 0.9 g NaCl/100 mL water. It contains 154 mmol sodium/L; no potassium chloride is added. This concentration makes it isotonic with plasma.

A one molar (1 mol/L) solution of NaCl would contain 58.5 g (1 mol) NaCl. In cases of hypovolaemia, intravenous colloid may be given as well as crystalloid to replace electrolytes.

1.43 Chronic vomiting   Answers: B D E

Patients with chronic vomiting tend to lose:

- large volumes of water
- hydrochloric acid (gastric acid in the stomach)
- $NaCl/K^+$.

This results in metabolic alkalosis, with a rise in blood pH. It is also known as hypochloraemic alkalosis. Continuous nasal gastric aspiration has the same effect.

The patient becomes dehydrated and sodium is depleted. In the compensatory mechanism, the kidney acts to conserve Na^+ in exchange for K^+ and H^+. This is paradoxical aciduria because of the following:

- H^+ is being lost despite the presence of an alkalosis.
- Hypokalaemia occurs because K^+ is lost in the vomit.
- K^+ is lost in the urine with H^+.
- Alkalosis causes K^+ to enter the cells.

1.44 Wound healing   Answers: A E

Wound healing depends on:

- A good blood supply
- Good apposition of tissues
- Tension-free edges.

It is enhanced by a good nutritional state. The following are the detrimental factors:

- Infection: local or distant – bacterial proteolytic enzymes break down healing tissues
- Foreign body, eg suture material
- Devitalised tissue: due to poor blood supply
- Haematoma: prevents good blood supply at the wound edges
- Tension
- Malnutrition: especially zinc and vitamin C deficiencies
- Trauma
- Metabolic diseases, eg diabetes mellitus
- Drugs, eg cytotoxics and steroids.

1.45 Nutritional problems post-gastrectomy   Answers: A C D E

With any operation, postoperative complications should be considered under the headings of 'early', 'intermediate' and 'late', with regard to the general and more specific complications of any particular operation. Nutritional problems after a gastrectomy take several months to develop. They include:

- **Dumping syndrome**:
  - as food passes rapidly through to the small bowel, the osmotic gradient draws water into the lumen; hypovolaemia occurs and blood pressure falls; the patient becomes pale, cold and clammy
  - as carbohydrate-rich foods enter the small bowel rapidly, insulin secretion increases; when no further carbohydrate is present a rebound hypoglycaemia results
- **Diarrhoea**: this is a result of 'blind loop syndrome'; in the polya type gastrectomy, a blind-ending loop of duodenum harbours bacteria. Bacterial overgrowth then results in diarrhoea and malabsorption. Diarrhoea may be severe and episodic
- **Vomiting**: the result of overfilling of the stomach. Sometimes bilious vomiting occurs before a meal as bile refluxes into the stomach remnant
- **Weight loss**: the result of vomiting/diarrhoea and poor appetite (because there is no stomach, there is no reservoir)
- **Vitamin B$_{12}$ deficiency:** loss of gastric intrinsic factor results in malabsorption of vitamin B$_{12}$. This causes a macrocytic megaloblastic anaemia. It takes between about 3 months and several years to develop as body stores are used up.
- **Iron deficiency anaemia**: normally the acid pH of the stomach increases iron absorption in the Fe^{3+} state. Therefore, reduced iron absorption results in iron deficiency anaemia.
- **Osteomalacia** as a result of malabsorption of calcium and vitamin D. Also the acid pH of the stomach reduces calcium absorption.
- **Steatorrhoea**: this is caused by poor mixing of food and enzymes, reduced pancreatic output and inactivation of enzymes in the afferent loops.

Other complications include the following:

- A feeling of fullness (the patient needs to eat small amounts of food frequently)
- Gastric outlet obstruction
- Ulceration in the gastric remnant (rare)
- Tumour in the gastric remnant.

1.46 Horner syndrome   Answers: B C E

The features of Horner syndrome are ptosis, miosis, anhidrosis and enophthalmos. Horner syndrome is the result of damage at the sympathetic nerves of the head and neck. The nerves involved are from T1 and its postganglionic connections, which synapse in the cervical ganglia. Interruption of the sympathetic nerve supply causes the following:

- The pupil to constrict
- Blood vessels to dilate – vasodilatation
- Reduced sweating
- Drooping of levator palpebrae superioris: this muscle of the eyelid is supplied by sympathetic nerves as well as the third cranial nerve. Interruption of sympathetic nerve function results in partial ptosis.

The following are causes of Horner syndrome:

- Brachial plexus injury
- Cervical sympathectomy – iatrogenic
- Lung tumours, ie Pancoast's tumour in the apex of the lung
- Brain lesions
- Syringomyelia or spinal cord lesions
- Carotid artery aneurysm
- Tumours in the neck.

1.47 Medial meniscus tear   Answers: A B C D E

Medial meniscus tears occur more frequently than lateral tears because the medial meniscus is attached to the capsule of the knee joint. This makes it less mobile and trauma is more likely to result in a tear.

If the cartilage then becomes jammed between the articular surfaces of the tibia and those of the femur, and 'locking' of the knee is felt, full extension of the knee is not possible. Full flexion is still possible.

The patient may complain that the knee 'gives way'. The history is usually of a twisting injury resulting in pain and swelling as a result of recurrent effusions, which may be haemarthrosis. In long-standing cases quadriceps wasting occurs. Investigations include arthroscopy or MRI.

Treatment:

- Conservative: the leg is put in plaster with the knee extended for 3–4 weeks
- Surgical: this can be done at arthroscopy, eg suturing or partial meniscectomy.

1.48 Neuromuscular blockers   Answer: E

Muscle relaxants are often used during surgery. Neuromuscular blockers are of two types:

1. Competitive inhibitors (eg tubocurarine, pancuronium, atracuronium and vecuronium). These agents are reversible: they act by competing with acetylcholine for the receptor site. Remember that the neurotransmitter at the neuromuscular junction is acetylcholine acting on muscarinic receptors. Increasing the concentration of tubocurarine, for example, displaces acetylcholine, and vice versa. Their action is terminated by the use of an anticholinesterase (eg neostigmine).
2. Depolarising blockers (eg suxamethonium). This agent is irreversible. Its initial action is to cause stimulation and hence muscle fasciculation may be seen. Patients often complain of muscular pain after an operation in which suxamethonium has been administered. Suxamethonium has a rapid onset and is short acting, and is normally metabolised by pseudocholinesterase. Note that some patients have a deficiency of this enzyme and in these cases the effects may be devastating. The deficiency is often familial and therefore a family history is very important.

1.49 Carcinoma of the stomach   Answers: B C D E

Carcinoma of the stomach is usually an adenocarcinoma. The aetiology is unknown. The associations include the following:

*   Genetics: first-degree relatives have an increased incidence
*   Blood group A (duodenal ulcers occur more commonly in blood group O)
*   Geographical (eg the incidence is higher in Japan, which is probably an environmental effect)
*   Social class: the incidence is higher in the lower social classes
*   Gastric mucosal atrophy predisposes to carcinoma (eg in gastritis and pernicious anaemia)
*   Polycyclic hydrocarbons and nitrosamines in the diet have been implicated
*   Cigarette smoking.

Carcinoma of the stomach is rare before the age of 50 years; it is more common in men than in women. Spread occurs locally, via the bloodstream and the lymphatics. Transcoelomic spread to the ovaries results in 'Krukenberg's tumours'.

1.50 Minimally invasive surgery

Answers: A B C

Minimally invasive surgery refers to those procedures that are performed with minimal access, eg laparoscopic surgery or ultrasound-guided abscess drainage. The incision is kept small. Laparoscopic surgery is commonly used for cholecystectomy and for hernia repair (keyhole surgery), but is now commonly used for appendicectomy, fundoplication, hemicolectomy, sympathectomy and nephrectomy.

The following are the advantages:

- Less operative trauma
- A reduction in postoperative complications
- Quicker recovery time and restoration of mobility
- Can be used for surgery in morbidly obese patients.

The following are the disadvantages:

- It takes longer (especially for inexperienced surgeons).
- It is expensive.
- Exposure is limited.
- It has its own inherent risks (eg bowel injury during introduction of the Veres needle or increased risk of bile duct injury during laparoscopic cholecystectomy).

1.51 Sarcoma

Answers: A B C D

Sarcoma is a Greek word meaning 'fleshy growth'. It refers to a malignant tumour arising in the tissues of mesenchymal origin, eg skeletal tissues. The suffix 'sarcoma' is used to denote malignancy, eg in bone the term used is 'osteosarcoma' and in smooth muscle it is 'leiomyosarcoma'. Osteosarcoma occurs most commonly in the metaphyses of the femur. The cause is mostly unknown. However, there are several associations:

- Inherited conditions (eg neurofibromatosis)
- Ionising radiation
- Scars from thermal and acid burns
- Kaposi's sarcoma, seen in AIDS.

Sarcomas tend to grow rapidly. Spread, as with any tumour, is:

- local
- via the bloodstream (the predominant route)
- via lymphatics.

Note that, in tumours such as those of the stomach, spread may occur via peritoneal fluids, ie transcoelomic spread.

Treatment of sarcomas is by a combination of surgery and radiotherapy. The use of adjuvant chemotherapy is controversial.

1.52 Prostate carcinoma   Answers: A C D E

Carcinoma of the prostate is the most common malignant condition in men aged over 65 years. A patient may present with the following:

- No symptoms
- Bladder outflow obstruction, ie hesitancy, poor stream, frequency, nocturia, post-micturition dribbling
- Manifestations of spread (see below).

The following are the modes of spread:

- **Local spread**: this involves local tissue, especially the rectum, and may result in a stricture. Rectal examination should be performed in all these patients. Local spread may cause a major DVT of the lower limbs by obstructing venous return.
- **Distant spread**: via the bloodstream, especially to the pelvis and vertebrae; lesions are typically sclerotic. Patients present with bone pain or pathological fractures. The rate of growth depends on testosterone concentration.

Treatment:

- Hormonal manipulation: orchidectomy – oestrogen
- Luteinising hormone-releasing hormone (LHRH)
- Anti-androgens, eg cyproterone acetate (CPA)
- Transurethral resection of the prostate – for early tumours
- Radiotherapy.

When describing the pathology of a condition use the mnemonic:

In A Surgeon's Gown A Physician May Make Some Terribly Clever Progress:

In	Incidence
A	Age
Surgeon's	Sex
Gown	Geography
A	Aetiology
Physician	Predisposition
May	Macroscopic features
Make	Microscopic features
Some	Spread
Terribly	Treatment
Clever	Complications
Progress	Prognosis

1.53 Postoperative complications

Answers: C E

Postoperative complications are best organised under the headings 'early', 'intermediate' and 'late':

- **Early**: up to 24 hours:
  - atelectasis/respiratory distress
  - reactionary haemorrhage
  - urinary retention.
- **Intermediate**: second day to 2 weeks:
  - lungs – atelectasis, infection, pulmonary embolism
  - bladder – urinary retention, UTI
  - legs – DVT
  - wound – infection, dehiscence, delayed haemorrhage.
- **Late**: weeks later:
  - wound dehiscence
  - incisional hernia
  - recurrent condition.

These are general complications. Further consideration needs to be given to the complications associated with specific operations, eg anastomotic leak in bowel surgery, nutritional complications after gastrectomy, or paralytic ileus and subphrenic abscesses after abdominal surgery.

1.54 Gas gangrene

Answers: B C

Gas gangrene develops when there is wound infection with *Clostridium perfringens*, a Gram-positive rod found in soil. It is an obligate anaerobe and therefore proliferates under anaerobic conditions. The organisms produce exotoxins that destroy tissue and result in necrosis. This produces gases within the tissues that can be felt as 'crepitus'. Tissue destruction is rapid, initially blackening the skin, which breaks down and becomes purulent. Application of antiseptic solutions such as iodine alone is not curative, but is used to clean wounds and prevent further infection.

Treatment is by the following:

- Excision of all necrotic tissue: the wound should be left open to allow drainage and not closed with sutures; dressing packs arc used to facilitate healing from inside out
- Intravenous benzylpenicillin: should be given prophylactically in injury or before amputation of a limb
- Hyperbaric oxygen therapy
- Antitoxin administration.

1.55 Benign breast change   Answers: A E

Benign breast change is a benign disorder of the breast in which there is an abnormal response of tissue growth to the hormonal cycle. It may represent the extreme end of a normal range. It is not pre-cancerous but cancer may coexist and hence be misdiagnosed. Benign breast change (also called fibrocystic disease or painful nodularity) presents with:

- one or more areas of lumpiness
- cysts
- diffuse nodularity
- pain or tenderness.

These changes tend to occur in a cyclical fashion. The treatment is as follows:

- Reassurance
- Lumpectomy for painful discrete lumps
- Mastectomy: very rare and only in severe debilitating cases.

1.56 Abdominal aortic aneurysm   Answers: A C

An aneurysm is a localised dilatation of an artery involving all the layers of the wall. It may be fusiform or saccular. The most common cause is atherosclerosis.

Other causes include:

- congenital aneurysms
- trauma
- syphilis
- collagen diseases (eg Marfan syndrome or Ehlers–Danlos syndrome).

A genetic disposition has been found. The incidence is higher in men aged over 60 years; it is associated with hypertension and smoking. It may be asymptomatic or produce a pulsatile mass in the abdomen, with abdominal pain radiating to the back. 'Shock' can develop if a leak or rupture occurs.

Aneurysms are most frequently found in the abdominal aorta and below. They are usually below the renal arteries. Calcification along the arterial wall often allows visualisation on a plain abdominal film. Other useful investigations are ultrasonography, CT and aortography, which are used to assess size.

Size is monitored with serial ultrasound scans; elective surgery is indicated when the aortic diameter is > 5 cm, although this limit varies, depending on the fitness of the patient for surgery and the rate of expansion of the aneurysm. The risk of rupture increases with size and when symptoms occur. Surgery involves repair of the aneurysm with a prosthetic graft.

1.57 Nasogastric tube   Answers: C E

In severe head injury where there is loss of the gag reflex, the airway needs to be protected. This can be done with a cuffed endotracheal tube. Insertion of a NGT is contraindicated in basal skull fractures because there is a risk of pushing the tube into the brain.

In small or large bowel obstruction, the first line of treatment is 'drip and suck', ie intravenous fluid maintenance and suction of stomach contents via an NGT.

The NGT is put on free drainage with aspiration at regular intervals. This relieves vomiting, protects the airway and protects the dilated bowel from any further fluid and air. These conservative measures may be enough to relieve the obstruction. If not, surgery is required. Nasogastric aspiration is not useful in assessing upper gastrointestinal blood loss because a considerable amount of blood may be lost into the lumen and appear as melaena. A fine-bore NGT is used for enteral feeding.

1.58 Pleomorphic adenoma (mixed parotid tumour)   Answers: A D E

Pleomorphic adenoma is an adenoma of salivary glands. Typically it presents as a painless slow-growing mass in the parotid gland. It is a benign tumour. The capsule is incomplete and the tumour may penetrate surrounding tissue. It may then recur or undergo malignant transformation. Thus, enucleation is not enough for removal – excision is required.

At surgery, there is a risk of facial nerve damage because the facial nerve branches within the gland. Frey syndrome occurs when the parasympathetic secretomotor nerve fibres to the gland are divided and then regenerate in the skin. This causes sweating on stimulation of the salivary gland, ie 'gustatory sweating'.

1.59 Carcinoma of the oesophagus   Answers: A B D E

Most carcinomas of the oesophagus are squamous cell tumours occurring in the middle third of the oesophagus.

The risk factors are alcohol, smoking and diet (nitrosamines).

There is an association with structural abnormalities, eg achalasia, oesophageal webs, strictures, pharyngeal pouch and Barrett's oesophagus.

Plummer–Vinson syndrome consists of dysphagia (resulting from an oesophageal web) with iron deficiency anaemia and is associated with carcinoma of the oesophagus.

1.60 Acute cholecystitis – treatment   **Answers: A B C D**

Uncomplicated acute cholecystitis will resolve with conservative treatment, ie bed rest, intravenous fluids, intravenous antibiotics and analgesia. Cholecystectomy may be performed early or late.

A laparoscopic or open technique may be used.

In the acute phase, laparoscopic surgery can be performed within 24–48 hours. Later, adhesions with inflammation and infection can make surgery difficult, and it is best left until after inflammation has settled.

Cholecystectomy is then performed 6–8 weeks after the acute episode, with tests for liver function to ensure that there is no biliary obstruction.

BEST OF FIVE AND MULTIPLE CHOICE QUESTIONS PAPER 2

60 questions: time allowed 2½ hours

Best of Five Questions
Mark your answers with a tick (True) in the box provided.

2.1   **A 17-year-old woman is admitted surgically with acute onset lower abdominal pain. On examination she has a tender left iliac fossa. What is the most appropriate next test?**

❑   A   Ultrasonography of the abdomen
❑   B   Gynaecological opinion
❑   C   Proctoscopy
❑   D   Laparoscopy
❑   E   Pregnancy test (β-hCG)

2.2   **A 34-year-old man with inflammatory bowel disease undergoes emergency surgery, involving resection of a portion of his bowel. At the clinicopathological conference, the histological findings of the operative sample are discussed. Which of the following features is most suggestive of Crohn's disease?**

❑   A   Crypt abscesses
❑   B   Mucosal inflammation
❑   C   Disease limited to the large bowel
❑   D   Transmural inflammation
❑   E   Continuous portions of disease

2.3   A 46-year-old solicitor complains of right upper quadrant pain
       and has deranged liver function tests (LFTs). Ultrasonography of
       the abdomen demonstrated a dilated common bile duct. He
       proceeds to endoscopic retrograde cholangiopancreatography
       (ERCP). While observing the procedure, the consultant asks you
       the location of the ampulla of Vater, which is cannulated during
       the procedure. Where does the ampulla of Vater enter the bowel?

- [ ] A   Jejunum
- [ ] B   Ascending duodenum (fourth part)
- [ ] C   Descending (second part) duodenum
- [ ] D   Inferior (third part) duodenum
- [ ] E   Superior (first part)

2.4   A 34-year-old, nutritionally deplete patient requires insertion of a
       nasogastric tube (NGT) to commence enteral feeding. What is the
       best precaution to take before starting the feeding regimen?

- [ ] A   Aspirate 10 mL from tube and inspect
- [ ] B   Insert 50 mL of air and auscultate over the stomach
- [ ] C   Aspirate 10 mL and check pH
- [ ] D   Chest radiograph
- [ ] E   Abdominal radiograph

2.5   A 54-year-old woman is admitted with left loin pain and
       haematuria. On examination she is tender in the left loin. A CT-
       KUB is performed. A left renal tract calculus is observed. What is
       the most common location of renal tract calculi?

- [ ] A   Renal pelvis
- [ ] B   Mid-ureter
- [ ] C   Vesicoureteric junction
- [ ] D   Pelvicoureteric junction
- [ ] E   Bladder

2.6   You are observing the repair of an inguinal hernia for the first
       time. The consultant asks you what forms the roof of the inguinal
       canal. The roof of the inguinal canal is formed by:

☐ A   The aponeurosis of the external oblique
☐ B   The lacunar ligament
☐ C   The reflected inguinal ligament
☐ D   The union of the transversalis fascia with the inguinal ligament
☐ E   The arched fibres of internal oblique and transversus abdominis

2.7   **While performing a cholecystectomy, the consultant ligates the cystic artery. The cystic artery supplying the gallbladder is usually a branch of:**

☐ A   The gastroduodenal artery
☐ B   The right gastric artery
☐ C   The hepatic proper artery
☐ D   The right hepatic artery
☐ E   The left hepatic artery

2.8   **A 36-year-old man with a tumour of the left submandibular gland proceeded to surgery. During surgery on the left submandibular gland the lingual nerve is injured. Postoperatively, the patient will complain of:**

☐ A   Deviation of the tongue to the right
☐ B   Deviation of the tongue to the left
☐ C   Loss of taste sensation over the anterior two-thirds of the left side of the tongue
☐ D   Loss of taste sensation over the posterior third of the left side of the tongue
☐ E   Loss of general sensation over the posterior third of the left side of the tongue

2.9   **A 22-year-old woman slipped and fell on her left hand. She sustained injury to her left anatomical snuffbox. An injury involving the anatomical snuffbox is likely to damage:**

☐ A   The radial nerve
☐ B   The median nerve
☐ C   The radial artery
☐ D   The ulnar nerve
☐ E   The ulnar artery

2.10   **A 50-year-old man with advanced cancer of the stomach complains of hoarseness. On clinical examination he has enlarged deep cervical lymph nodes. The hoarse voice is a result of enlarged nodes pressing on:**

❑   A   The recurrent laryngeal branch of vagus
❑   B   The external branch of the superior laryngeal nerve
❑   C   The internal branch of the superior laryngeal nerve
❑   D   The nerve to the cricothyroid muscle
❑   E   The pharyngeal branch of the glossopharyngeal nerve

2.11   **A 46-year-old African woman is to undergo splenectomy for an enlarged spleen. The consultant warns his registrar that, while performing splenectomy, he must identify the tail of pancreas to avoid postoperative pancreatic fistula. At the time of splenectomy, the tail of pancreas must be identified in:**

❑   A   The transverse mesocolon
❑   B   The gastrocolic ligament
❑   C   The gastrosplenic ligament
❑   D   The phrenicocolic ligament
❑   E   The splenorenal ligament

2.12   **A 22-year-old woman has an enlarged lymph node in the posterior triangle of her neck. The consultant asks you to define the boundaries of the posterior triangle of the neck. The posterior triangle of the neck is bounded by:**

❑   A   The anterior border of the sternocleidomastoid muscle, inferior border of the mandible and anterior midline of the neck
❑   B   The anterior borders of both sternocleidomastoid muscles, inferior border of the mandible and suprasternal notch of the manubrium
❑   C   The posterior border of the sternocleidomastoid muscle, clavicle and anterior border of the trapezius muscle
❑   D   The anterior borders of both trapezius muscles, occipital bone and posterior midline of the neck
❑   E   Both bellies of the digastric muscle and inferior border of the mandible

2.13   A 34-year-old woman with a carotid body tumour proceeded to surgery. While exposing the internal carotid artery in the carotid triangle to access the tumour, the surgeon must avoid a vital structure that lies anteromedial to the internal carotid artery. This vital structure is:

- ❑ A   The internal jugular vein
- ❑ B   The vagus nerve
- ❑ C   The glossopharyngeal nerve
- ❑ D   The hypoglossal nerve
- ❑ E   The external carotid artery

2.14   A 24-year-old man was stabbed with a broken piece of glass in his neck during a bar fight. On arrival in A&E he was examined and the spinal accessory nerve (cranial nerve or CN XI) was found to be injured. Damage to the spinal accessory nerve (CN XI) will result in weakness and atrophy of:

- ❑ A   Rhomboid major
- ❑ B   Trapezius
- ❑ C   Teres minor
- ❑ D   Levator scapulae
- ❑ E   Splenius capitis

2.15   A 36-year-old man presents with a trophic ulcer over the ball of the big toe of his right foot. Which of the following conditions is least likely to be diagnosed in this patient?

- ❑ A   Tuberculosis (TB)
- ❑ B   Chronic vasospasm
- ❑ C   Syringomyelia
- ❑ D   Diabetes
- ❑ E   Spina bifida

Multiple Choice Questions

Mark your answers with a tick (True) or a cross (False) in the box provided. Leave the box blank for 'Don't know'. Do not look at the answers until you have completed the whole question paper.

2.16   Avascular necrosis:

- ☐ A   Is a typical complication of fracture of the scaphoid bone
- ☐ B   Is a typical complication of fracture of the femoral shaft
- ☐ C   May result from venous occlusion
- ☐ D   Presents early with pain
- ☐ E   May result from arterial occlusion

2.17   A man sustains a laceration to the wrist from a broken glass, dividing his radial artery. The following are appropriate at presentation:

- ☐ A   Radiograph
- ☐ B   Pressure dressing
- ☐ C   Tourniquet
- ☐ D   Tetanus prophylaxis
- ☐ E   Nerve conduction studies to detect median nerve damage

2.18   Warfarin:

- ☐ A   Must be replaced by heparin before surgery
- ☐ B   May be reversed by protamine sulphate
- ☐ C   May be reversed by vitamin K
- ☐ D   Is monitored by prothrombin time, reported as the international normalised ratio (INR)
- ☐ E   Is mandatory after insertion of a prosthetic heart valve

2.19   Deep vein thrombosis (DVT):

- ☐ A   Usually results from incompetent superficial veins
- ☐ B   Is prevented by heparin
- ☐ C   Is treated with heparin
- ☐ D   Is more common in malignancy
- ☐ E   Is diagnosed by duplex scanning

2.20   Hoarseness of the voice:

☐ A   Is common in myxoedema
☐ B   May be a sign of anaplastic thyroid carcinoma
☐ C   May be a feature of laryngeal carcinoma
☐ D   Usually occurs with pharyngeal pouch
☐ E   Is severe in bilateral recurrent laryngeal nerve palsy

2.21   Which of the following statements are true?

☐ A   Diverticulosis coli results from a congenital malformation
☐ B   Diverticular disease is pre-malignant
☐ C   Diverticulosis causes rectal bleeding
☐ D   The diagnosis of diverticulitis is made on ultrasound scan of the abdomen
☐ E   Pneumaturia may be caused by diverticulitis

2.22   In gastric ulceration:

☐ A   Malignant change eventually supervenes
☐ B   An hour-glass stomach may occur
☐ C   Excess acid secretion is the main cause
☐ D   Carbenoxolone sodium may promote healing
☐ E   The majority of benign ulcers are situated in the greater curvature

2.23   Familial adenomatous polyposis:

☐ A   May be inherited as an autosomal dominant condition
☐ B   Is pre-malignant
☐ C   Occurs in severe ulcerative colitis
☐ D   May cause electrolyte disturbance
☐ E   May be asymptomatic

2.24   Crohn's disease:

☐ A   Is familial
☐ B   Is a malignant condition
☐ C   Has Reed–Sternberg cells which are pathognomonic
☐ D   Produces caseating granulomas
☐ E   Is a transmural disease of the small bowel only

2.25 **Symptoms of mesenteric embolus include:**

- ❑ A Rebound tenderness
- ❑ B Melaena
- ❑ C Hypotension
- ❑ D Visible peristalsis
- ❑ E Haematemesis

2.26 **Constipation may be caused by:**

- ❑ A Opiates
- ❑ B Aluminium hydroxide preparations
- ❑ C Hypothyroidism
- ❑ D Diabetes insipidus
- ❑ E Lactulose

2.27 **With regard to haemorrhoids:**

- ❑ A Thrombosis is a recognised complication
- ❑ B They can be treated with band ligation
- ❑ C First-degree piles are best treated with haemorrhoidectomy
- ❑ D They predispose to carcinoma
- ❑ E Strangulation can be treated with haemorrhoidectomy

2.28 **Symptoms of a strangulated femoral hernia include:**

- ❑ A Irreducibility
- ❑ B Overlying redness
- ❑ C Tenderness
- ❑ D Diarrhoea
- ❑ E A fluid thrill on coughing

2.29 **Recognised modes of presentation of gallstones include:**

- ❑ A Dysphagia
- ❑ B Abdominal pain
- ❑ C Shoulder tip pain
- ❑ D Small bowel obstruction
- ❑ E Tenesmus

2.30   Features of hydatid cysts in the liver include:

- ❑ A   Menorrhagia
- ❑ B   Calcification on a plain abdominal radiograph
- ❑ C   Haemoptysis
- ❑ D   Anaphylaxis
- ❑ E   Jaundice

2.31   A swelling presenting just below the angle of the mandible in a 30-year-old man may be:

- ❑ A   A pharyngeal pouch
- ❑ B   An enlarged lymph node
- ❑ C   A thyroglossal cyst
- ❑ D   A carotid body tumour
- ❑ E   Ectopic thyroid tissue

2.32   The incidence of breast cancer is higher in women who:

- ❑ A   Have already had breast cancer
- ❑ B   Are young
- ❑ C   Have breast-fed their children
- ❑ D   Are obese
- ❑ E   Have a family history of ovarian carcinoma

2.33   A patient presents with a large swelling confined to the scrotum. It is transilluminable and the testis can be felt separately. The diagnosis may be:

- ❑ A   A hydrocele
- ❑ B   An inguinal hernia
- ❑ C   A hydrocele of the cord
- ❑ D   An epididymal cyst
- ❑ E   Epididymal TB

2.34   Acute renal failure after major abdominal surgery may be caused by:

- ❑ A   Hypotension during the operation
- ❑ B   A haemolytic transfusion reaction
- ❑ C   Gram-negative septicaemia
- ❑ D   Blood loss
- ❑ E   Fluid overload

2.35 After a head injury, an extradural haematoma:

☐ A Can be confidently excluded if the patient is conscious
☐ B Causes dilatation of the contralateral pupil at an early stage
☐ C Causes deterioration in the level of consciousness
☐ D Is always associated with a fractured skull
☐ E Is characteristically associated with an increased heart rate and blood pressure

2.36 An undescended testis:

☐ A Should be brought into the scrotum after the age of 10 years
☐ B Is rarely associated with an inguinal hernia
☐ C Is prone to malignant change
☐ D Is more likely to undergo torsion than a normal testis
☐ E Means that the patient will be sterile

2.37 A varicocele:

☐ A May be treated by sclerotherapy
☐ B Is usually right sided
☐ C Is associated with a renal tumour
☐ D Can be treated by embolisation
☐ E May cause pain

2.38 Raynaud's phenomenon may be associated with:

☐ A Carcinoma of the oesophagus
☐ B Pernicious anaemia
☐ C Atheroma of the subclavian artery
☐ D Carcinoma of the testis
☐ E Rheumatoid arthritis

2.39 Complications of acute pancreatitis include:

☐ A Carcinoma of the pancreas
☐ B Stones in the common bile duct
☐ C Pseudocyst formation
☐ D Obstruction of the transverse colon
☐ E Fat embolus

2.40   Rodent ulcers:

❏   A   Are squamous cell carcinomas
❏   B   Are basal cell carcinomas
❏   C   Occur only on the face
❏   D   Show epithelial pearls
❏   E   Metastasise via the bloodstream

2.41   Tetany is a recognised complication of:

❏   A   Metabolic alkalosis
❏   B   Thyroidectomy
❏   C   A deep dirty wound of the foot
❏   D   Overbreathing
❏   E   Paralytic ileus

2.42   An acutely infected, ingrowing toenail may be treated by:

❏   A   Keller's osteotomy
❏   B   Amputation of the toe
❏   C   Wedge excision of the nail and nail bed
❏   D   Antibiotics
❏   E   Nail avulsion

2.43   In a man aged 50 years with a 3-year history of indigestion, features of the management of 1 L haematemesis should be the following:

❏   A   A barium meal should be performed within 24 hours
❏   B   Gastroscopy must be postponed for 48 hours after the last episode of bleeding
❏   C   In view of the history an operation should follow initial resuscitation
❏   D   Blood transfusion should be started if the haemoglobin is < 9 g/dL
❏   E   A careful watch should be kept on the pulse, blood pressure and central venous pressure

2.44 A pilonidal sinus is:

- ❏ A A sinus containing hair
- ❏ B A fistula *in ano* containing hair
- ❏ C An abscess in a hair-bearing area
- ❏ D A sinus that commonly occurs in the natal cleft
- ❏ E Often associated with a number of subcutaneous tracks

2.45 Malignant melanoma:

- ❏ A Is not always pigmented
- ❏ B May arise from junctional naevi
- ❏ C May itch
- ❏ D Has metastases in regional lymph nodes that are very effectively treated by external radiotherapy
- ❏ E Regresses after hypophysectomy

2.46 Carotid artery stenosis:

- ❏ A May be asymptomatic
- ❏ B Causes amaurosis fugax
- ❏ C Causes vomiting
- ❏ D Causes transient ischaemic attacks
- ❏ E Is treated with carotid endarterectomy if the stenosis is 20%

2.47 In a compound fracture:

- ❏ A The bone is broken into many fragments
- ❏ B The overlying soft tissues are broken, with free communication to the exterior
- ❏ C Patients should be given appropriate antibiotic cover
- ❏ D Surgical fixation of the fracture is contraindicated
- ❏ E The bone is broken in two or more places

2.48 Ranitidine:

- ❏ A Acts by blocking histamine receptors
- ❏ B Is an H_1-receptor antagonist
- ❏ C Is used to prevent stress ulcers
- ❏ D Can be given intravenously
- ❏ E Should be avoided in the first 12 h after a gastrointestinal bleed

2.49 **The following are more likely to occur in ulcerative colitis than in Crohn's disease:**

- ❏ A Rectal bleeding
- ❏ B Abdominal mass
- ❏ C Steatorrhoea
- ❏ D Rectal involvement
- ❏ E Fistulae

2.50 **Dupuytren's contracture is:**

- ❏ A More common in men than in women
- ❏ B Associated with alcoholic cirrhosis of the liver
- ❏ C Associated with underlying malignancy
- ❏ D Transmitted as an autosomal recessive condition
- ❏ E Associated with renal failure

2.51 **A closed fracture of the femoral shaft:**

- ❏ A May be complicated by fat embolism
- ❏ B May require blood transfusion
- ❏ C Requires tetanus immunisation
- ❏ D May require intramedullary nailing
- ❏ E Will have healed fully within 6 weeks

2.52 **Some 18 hours after an operation it is noticed that a patient has not passed urine. Which of the following would always be appropriate?**

- ❏ A Intravenous infusion of 10% mannitol
- ❏ B Injection of 20 mg furosemide (frusemide)
- ❏ C Catheterisation of the bladder
- ❏ D Examination of the bladder
- ❏ E Renal dose of dopamine

2.53 **'Cellulitis' is a term used to describe:**

- ❏ A Death of liver cells in association with circulating toxins
- ❏ B Inflammation surrounding a malignant tumour
- ❏ C Spreading infection in the subcutaneous tissue
- ❏ D TB involving the skin
- ❏ E An abscess occurring in a surgical wound

2.54   Salivary duct calculi:

☐ A   Are more common in the parotid duct than in the submandibular duct
☐ B   Are usually radio-opaque
☐ C   Cause pain on eating
☐ D   Can be confirmed with sialography
☐ E   Are usually treated by surgical removal of the gland

2.55   Cancer of the stomach:

☐ A   Has a 5-year survival rate of more than 40%
☐ B   Is most common in the antrum
☐ C   Metastasises to lymph nodes
☐ D   May present with an abdominal mass
☐ E   Is treated by gastrectomy

2.56   Ureteric calculi:

☐ A   Produce pain that is colicky in nature
☐ B   Should routinely be surgically removed
☐ C   Are predominantly 'triple phosphate'
☐ D   Can be treated by lithotripsy
☐ E   Predispose to transitional cell carcinoma of the ureter

2.57   The normal metabolic response to trauma is characterised by:

☐ A   An increase in lean body mass
☐ B   Antidiuretic hormone (ADH) release
☐ C   Gluconeogenesis
☐ D   A positive nitrogen balance
☐ E   Potassium loss

2.58   The passage of bright red blood with faeces may be caused by:

☐ A   A thrombosed haemorrhoid
☐ B   Anal fissure
☐ C   Ischiorectal abscess
☐ D   Carcinoma of the colon at the hepatic flexure
☐ E   Haemorrhoids

2.59   Staging of breast tumours:

☐   A   Assesses extent of spread
☐   B   Indicates prognosis
☐   C   Does not take nodal involvement into account
☐   D   Is performed by mammography
☐   E   Is of use only in women

2.60   Hypocalcaemia may occur in:

☐   A   Multiple myeloma
☐   B   Parathyroid adenoma
☐   C   Acute pancreatitis
☐   D   Gallstones
☐   E   Post-thyroidectomy

———————————— **END** ————————————

**Go over your answers until your time is up. Correct answers
and teaching notes are overleaf.**

BEST OF FIVE AND MULTIPLE CHOICE QUESTIONS PAPER 2
Answers

The correct answer options for each question are given below.

2.1	E	2.31	B D
2.2	D	2.32	A D E
2.3	C	2.33	C D
2.4	D	2.34	A B C D
2.5	C	2.35	C
2.6	E	2.36	C D
2.7	D	2.37	C D E
2.8	C	2.38	C E
2.9	C	2.39	C E
2.10	A	2.40	B
2.11	E	2.41	A B D
2.12	C	2.42	C D E
2.13	E	2.43	D E
2.14	B	2.44	A D E
2.15	A	2.45	A B C
2.16	A C E	2.46	A B D
2.17	A B D	2.47	B C
2.18	C D E	2.48	A C D
2.19	B C D E	2.49	A D
2.20	B C D	2.50	A B
2.21	E	2.51	A B D
2.22	B D	2.52	C D
2.23	A B D E	2.53	C
2.24	None correct	2.54	B C D
2.25	A B C	2.55	B C D E
2.26	A B C	2.56	A D
2.27	A B E	2.57	B C E
2.28	A B C	2.58	B E
2.29	B C D	2.59	A B
2.30	B C D E	2.60	C E

BEST OF FIVE AND MULTIPLE CHOICE QUESTIONS PAPER 2
Answers and Teaching Notes

2.1   E: Pregnancy test (β-hCG)

Always consider the possibility of gynaecological problems in a woman of child-bearing age with abdominal pain.

One should consider whether this patient may be pregnant and the cause of pain is an ectopic pregnancy. Part of the clinical history should be asking the date of the patient's last menstrual period (LMP) and about a sexual history. If there is any ongoing clinical concern a pregnancy test should be performed.

β Human chorionic gonadotrophin (β-hCG) may be measured in both the urine and the serum.

2.2   D: Transmural inflammation

Inflammatory bowel disease is a term that encompasses ulcerative colitis and Crohn's disease.

Ulcerative colitis is a disease exclusive to the large bowel, whereas Crohn's disease may involve any part of the gastrointestinal tract from mouth to anus. It may affect only the large bowel, when it is termed Crohn's colitis. This can be difficult to distinguish clinically from ulcerative colitis. Histopathology of surgical specimens then holds the diagnostic key.

Histopathological features of inflammatory bowel disease

	Crohn's disease	Ulcerative colitis
Inflammation	Transmural	Mucosal
Crypt abscesses	No	Yes
Rose thorn (deep) Ulcers:	Yes	No
Lesions	Skip	Continuous
Granulomas	Yes	No

2.3   C: Descending (second part) duodenum

The small intestine is composed of the duodenum, jejunum and ileum. The duodenum is divided into four parts: ascending, descending, inferior and superior. The duodenum is C shaped, the first part often being referred to as the duodenal cap. The confluence of the common bile duct and pancreatic duct enters the descending (second) part of the duodenum as the ampulla of Vater (major duodenal papilla). The side-viewing aspect of the ERCP endoscope is used to cannulate the ampulla of Vater, allowing access to the biliary tree.

2.4   D: Chest radiograph

The placement of an NGT has two main indications:

1. For enteral feeding/medication administration
2. For decompression of the stomach.

A fine-bore tube is used for the former and a larger-calibre (Salem sump) tube is used for the latter.

Although all the above methods listed are potentially possible methods of confirmation of correct NGT placement, the most correct is a check chest radiograph. If an NGT is being used purely for aspiration/decompression, aspiration options A–C may suffice. If feeding is to be started it is ESSENTIAL that a chest radiograph be performed. Should NGT feeding start with it incorrectly placed in a bronchus, the outcome may be fatal.

2.5   C: Vesicoureteric junction

CT-KUB (computed tomography of the kidney, ureter and bladder) is the first-line imaging modalities in most centres for patients with renal colic, although intravenous urography (IVU) is still used. A plain abdominal radiograph is of limited use in acute renal colic, but may be used to monitor a known radio-opaque calculus.

Renal calculi come in various types:

- Calcium oxalate (majority)
- Triple phosphate
- Uric acid
- Cystine
- Xanthine.

The three most common locations (from proximal to distal) within the renal tract are:

1. Pelvicoureteric junction
2. Within the ureter at the pelvic brim
3. Vesicoureteric junction (the most common).

2.6   E: Arched fibres of internal oblique and transversus abdominis

The inguinal canal is an oblique canal about 4 cm long, slanting downwards and medially, and placed parallel with and a little above the inguinal ligament. It extends from the abdominal inguinal ring to the subcutaneous inguinal ring. It is bounded by the integument and superficial fascia in front, by the aponeurosis of the external oblique throughout its whole length, and by the internal oblique in its lateral third; behind, it is bounded by the reflected inguinal ligament, inguinal aponeurotic falx, transversalis fascia, extraperitoneal connective tissue and peritoneum; above (roof), it is bounded by the arched fibres of internal oblique and transversus abdominis, below (floor) by the union of the transversalis fascia with the inguinal ligament, and at its medial end by the lacunar ligament. The inguinal canal contains the spermatic cord and the ilioinguinal nerve in the male, and the round ligament of the uterus and the ilioinguinal nerve in the female.

2.7   D: Right hepatic artery

The cystic artery, usually a branch of the right hepatic, passes downwards and forwards along the neck of the gallbladder, and divides into two branches, one of which ramifies on the free surface, and the other on the attached surface of the gallbladder.

2.8   C: Loss of taste sensation over the anterior two-thirds of the left side of the tongue

The lingual nerve is one of the two terminal branches of the posterior division of the mandibular nerve. It is sensory to the anterior two-thirds of the tongue and floor of the mouth. However, the fibres of the chorda tympani (branch of facial nerve), which is secretomotor to the submandibular and sublingual salivary glands and gustatory to the anterior two-thirds of the tongue, are also distributed through the lingual nerve. Lingual nerve injury causing numbness, dysaesthesia, paraesthesia and dysgeusia, involving the anterior two-thirds of the tongue (on the same side), may complicate invasive dental and surgical therapies.

2.9   C: Radial artery

The anatomical snuffbox is a triangular depression on the lateral side of the wrist. It is seen best when the thumb is extended. It is bounded anteriorly by the tendons of abductor pollicis longus and extensor pollicis brevis, and posteriorly by the tendon of extensor pollicis longus. It is limited above by the styloid process of the radius. The floor of the snuffbox is formed by the scaphoid and the trapezium, and is crossed by the radial artery.

2.10   A: Recurrent laryngeal branch of vagus

Damage to the recurrent laryngeal nerve is one possible cause of hoarseness. The recurrent laryngeal nerve changes its name to the inferior laryngeal nerve at the level of the inferior border of the cricoid cartilage. The inferior laryngeal nerve goes on to innervate all the intrinsic muscles of the larynx except cricothyroideus. So, if this nerve innervating all the muscles of the larynx were damaged, a patient would have a hoarse voice. The external and internal branches of the superior laryngeal nerve innervate cricothyroid and the inferior pharyngeal constrictor, and provide secretomotor fibres to mucosal glands of the larynx above the vocal folds. The pharyngeal branch of the glossopharyngeal nerve provides sensory innervation to the pharynx.

2.11   E: Splenorenal ligament

The splenorenal ligament is the peritoneal structure that connects the spleen to the posterior abdominal wall over the left kidney. It also contains the tail of the pancreas.

The transverse mesocolon connects the transverse colon to the posterior abdominal wall. The gastrocolic ligament connects the greater curvature of the stomach with the transverse colon. The gastrosplenic ligament connects the greater curvature of the stomach with the hilum of the spleen. Finally, the phrenicolic ligament connects the splenic flexure of the colon to the diaphragm.

2.12   C: Posterior border of the sternocleidomastoid muscle, clavicle and anterior border of the trapezius muscle

The posterior triangle is bounded by sternocleidomastoid in front, and by the anterior margin of trapezius behind; its base is formed by the middle third of the clavicle, and its apex by the occipital bone. The space is crossed, about 2.5 cm above the clavicle, by the inferior belly of the omohyoid, which divides it into two triangles, an upper or occipital, and a lower or subclavian.

2.13 E: External carotid artery

The internal carotid artery supplies the anterior part of the brain, the eye and its appendages, and sends branches to the forehead and nose. In the neck the internal carotid begins at the bifurcation of the common carotid, opposite the upper border of the thyroid cartilage, and runs perpendicularly upwards, in front of the transverse processes of the upper three cervical vertebrae, to the carotid canal in the petrous portion of the temporal bone. It is comparatively superficial at its start, where it is contained in the carotid triangle, and lies behind and lateral to the external carotid, overlapped by sternocleidomastoid, and covered by the deep fascia, platysma and integument. It then passes beneath the parotid gland, being crossed by the hypoglossal nerve, the digastric and stylohyoid muscles, and the occipital and posterior auricular arteries.

2.14 B: Trapezius

The spinal accessory nerve exits from the jugular foramen and runs backwards in front of the internal jugular vein in 66.6% of cases, and behind it in 33.3%. The nerve then descends obliquely behind the digastric and stylohyoid to the upper part of sternocleidomastoid; it pierces this muscle and courses obliquely across the posterior triangle of the neck, to end in the deep surface of trapezius. As it traverses sternocleidomastoid, it gives several filaments to the muscle, and joins with branches from the second cervical nerve. In the posterior triangle it unites with the second and third cervical nerves, whereas beneath trapezius it forms a plexus with the third and fourth cervical nerves, and from this plexus fibres are distributed to the muscle.

2.15 A: TB

Trophic ulcers (*trophe* [Greek] = nutrition) are the result of an impairment of the nutrition of the tissues, which depends on an adequate blood supply and a properly functioning nerve supply. Ischemia and anaesthesia will therefore cause these ulcers. Thus, in the arm, chronic vasospasm and syringomyelia will cause ulceration of the tips of the fingers (painful and painless, respectively). In the leg, painful ischaemic ulcers occur around the ankle or on the dorsum of the foot. Neuropathic ulcers caused by anaesthesia (diabetic neuritis, spina bifida, tabes dorsalis, leprosy or a peripheral nerve injury) are often called perforating ulcers. Starting in a corn or bunion, they penetrate the foot, and suppuration may involve the bones and joints, and spread along fascial planes upwards, even involving the calf.

2.16 Avascular necrosis   Answers: A C E

Avascular necrosis of bone is caused by impaired blood supply, resulting in ischaemic damage to the bone. The causes are:

- trauma – damaged arterial supply or venous occlusion
- infection
- vasculitis
- sickle cell disease
- high-dose steroids.

Certain fractures are particularly susceptible to ischaemic necrosis, eg:

- femoral head and condyles
- head of humerus
- scaphoid, lunate, talus.

These rely on a main nutrient artery and have little collateral circulation.

Clinical features: the early stage is asymptomatic. Pain is usually the presenting symptom but occurs late when bone damage has occurred.

2.17 A man sustains a laceration to the wrist from broken glass, dividing his radial artery   Answers: A B D

The initial treatment involves management of the airway, breathing and circulation (ABC). Haemorrhage is best stopped in the acute phase by compression at the point of bleeding. A tourniquet is dangerous because it compromises the remaining circulation.

Radiographs are useful for detecting glass fragments, although not infallible. Tetanus prophylaxis is mandatory and tetanus immunoglobulin should be given if there has been no previous immunisation.

The median nerve may be damaged and the signs will suggest this. Nerve conduction studies are helpful after the acute injury.

Clinical features include the following:

- Motor function: loss of abduction of the thumb; later, the thenar eminence becomes wasted
- Sensory loss over the palmar aspect of the thumb and lateral two and a half fingers.

2.18 Warfarin   Answers: C D E

Warfarin is an anticoumarin. It is a vitamin K analogue and reduces production of the vitamin K clotting factors. Its effects are measured by prothrombin time (PT), represented as the INR. This is the ratio of measured PT to that of the normal population.

Anticoagulation is often reduced before surgery (to an INR of about 1.5). If there is a high risk of bleeding, warfarin is withheld for 3 days before surgery to reduce its effects, and substituted with heparin or fragmin, which is more controllable. Heparin has a shorter half-life and can be reversed quickly by protamine sulphate.

Patients on warfarin for atrial fibrillation need to omit only the dose before, and resume taking it after, surgery.

Patients with prosthetic heart valves, where the risk of thrombosis is high, require continuous anticoagulation. Patients with prosthetic heart valves are maintained on permanent oral warfarin anticoagulation. Patients with tissue (porcine) valves do not require anticoagulants.

2.19 Deep vein thrombosis (DVT)   Answers: B C D E

DVT is a postoperative complication. There is an increased risk in:

- elderly people
- immobile patients
- malignancy
- abdominal and pelvic surgery
- orthopaedic surgery
- prothrombotic blood disorders, eg protein C deficiency, protein S deficiency, antithrombin III deficiency and factor V Leiden.

Superficial vein incompetence may be a contributing factor but is not usually the cause.

Investigations include duplex scanning and phlebography. A blood test for D-dimers is helpful but has a high false-positive rate.

DVT is treated with anticoagulation. Fragmin injections are increasingly used in the community setting. Warfarin is a long-term alternative for patients who are at increased risk.

DVT prophylaxis is essential for surgical patients. It should include the following:

- Early mobilisation after surgery
- Intermittent pneumatic compression during surgery
- Compression stockings after surgery
- Subcutaneous heparin or fractionated low-molecular-weight heparin daily
- Avoidance of hormonal preparations that increase risk of thrombosis.

Aspirin has antiplatelet action and will reduce thrombosis. Treatment involves anticoagulation with intravenous heparin, compression stockings and then conversion to oral anticoagulation with warfarin.

2.20 Hoarseness of the voice   Answers: B C D

Myxoedema is hypothyroidism. It usually affects women aged over 50 years. The voice becomes deep and slow. Other features include:

- bradycardia
- constipation
- thick, coarse, dry skin
- thin hair.

In thyroid disease the vocal folds are affected when there is infiltration of the recurrent laryngeal nerves (RLNs). This occurs in thyroid carcinoma, especially anaplastic thyroid carcinoma. Laryngoscopy to check the vocal folds should be performed routinely in all patients before thyroid surgery.

Bilateral RLN palsy will cause loss of voice. Both vocal folds are then held in the neutral position, which causes respiratory difficulty.

The RLN supplies all the intrinsic laryngeal muscles except for the cricothyroid, which is supplied by the superior laryngeal nerve.

Laryngeal carcinoma may of course affect the voice directly. The left RLN may be affected in bronchial or oesophageal carcinoma.

Pharyngeal pouch causes dysphagia. The pouch arises at the junction of the pharynx and the oesophagus and consists of a mucosal outpouching between the inferior constrictor muscle and the cricopharyngeal muscle (Killian's dehiscence). Regurgitation of food may occur with aspiration. Food or acid reflux may cause hoarseness of the voice.

2.21 Diverticular disease   Answer: E

Diverticulosis coli is an acquired condition, caused by mucosa herniating through weak areas of muscle in the large bowel wall, after high intraluminal pressures from peristalsis. The sigmoid colon is the most commonly affected part, but diverticula may be present in any part of the colon. It is thought to be caused by the lack of fibre in the diet.

Diverticulosis refers to the asymptomatic condition.

Inflammation of a diverticulum (or several) is called 'diverticulitis', which is symptomatic. The common symptoms are:

- left iliac fossa pain
- fever
- rectal bleeding.

This leads to complications such as abscess formation, perforation, obstruction, and formation of adhesions, colovesical fistulae and strictures. A colovesical fistula presents with pneumaturia and cystitis.

Diverticular disease is not pre-malignant. Diagnosis of diverticular disease is best made on a barium enema or colonoscopy. Ultrasonography is useful to detect abscess formation.

A barium enema or colonoscopy is performed after the episode of acute inflammation has resolved to reduce the risk of perforation.

2.22 Gastric ulcers   Answers: B D

Most gastric ulcers occur on the lesser curve. The frequency increases with age and there is an association with blood group A. It is more common in lower socioeconomic classes. Acid secretion tends to be normal or low. The main problem is thought to be reduced mucosal resistance to acid (in contrast to duodenal ulcers where acid secretion is abnormally high).

Cigarette smoking is another association.

Helicobacter pylori is associated with both gastric and duodenal ulcers, and therefore eradication therapy plays an important role. This is based on 'triple therapy' with a proton pump inhibitor (PPI, eg omeprazole) and two antibiotics (amoxicillin and metronidazole).

Weight loss is a significant symptom in gastric ulceration because eating often causes pain, whereas in duodenal ulceration pain is often relieved by food.

Gastric ulceration may be benign or malignant. Whether benign ulcers progress to malignancy remains controversial.

2.23 Familial adenomatous polyposis   Answers: A B D E

Familial adenomatous polyposis (FAP) is an autosomal dominant inherited condition. It is characterised by multiple polyps throughout the colon and rectum. It develops during the teenage years, when it is initially asymptomatic and benign. Later, symptoms develop and patients present with a change in bowel habit, eg loose stools, rectal bleeding and mucus per rectum. Malignant change inevitably occurs within 20 years. Prophylactic surgery is the treatment of choice, with total colectomy and ileorectal anastomosis or pouch–anal anastomosis. In ulcerative colitis, inflammatory polyps may occur, but this is not the inherited condition FAP. Electrolyte disturbance occurs when there is considerable loss of mucus and blood per rectum.

2.24 Crohn's disease   Answer: None correct

The aetiology of Crohn's disease is unknown. There may be a genetic predisposition because there is sometimes a family history.

Pathology: Crohn's disease can occur anywhere along the gastrointestinal tract from the mouth to the anus. It is characterised by the following:

- Transmural involvement of the bowel, ie it affects the whole thickness of the wall
- Granuloma formation (non-caseating)
- Skip lesions, ie patchy involvement with normal areas in between
- Inflammation and oedema of the bowel wall
- Deep ulceration.

It is not a malignant condition.

Reed–Sternberg cells are seen in Hodgkin's disease.

2.25 Mesenteric embolus   Answers: A B C

Mesenteric ischaemia is a lack of blood supply to the mesentery. This may be caused by:

- embolus
- thrombosis
- reduced cardiac output (as a result of, for example, myocardial infarction)
- blocked venous drainage
- hypovolaemia.

In mesenteric embolus, oedema and inflammation of the bowel wall may result in rupture of blood vessels, causing haemorrhage into the bowel. The signs are:

- abdominal pain with rebound tenderness
- pyrexia
- dehydration
- vomiting

- white cell count (WCC) > 30 000/mm^3
- acidosis.

Abdominal signs are often mild and deceptive, even with extensive bowel damage. Paralytic ileus often occurs.

The signs of generalised peritonitis occur if there is perforation. About 90% of mesenteric emboli arise from the heart in association with atrial fibrillation. The extent of bowel affected depends on the site of final impaction.

2.26 Constipation   Answers: A B C

The causes of constipation are:

- drugs (eg opiates, iron, aluminium hydroxide preparations)
- hypothyroidism
- inactivity
- low-fibre diet
- faecal impaction
- bowel strictures (eg in diverticular disease or carcinoma).

'Absolute constipation' refers to the absence of flatus as well as faeces.

2.27 Haemorrhoids   Answers: A B E

See also the explanation to Question 1.28, Paper 1.

The management of haemorrhoids is as follows:

- **Conservative**: high-fibre diet, avoidance of straining and good anal hygiene.
- **Medical**: local anaesthetic agents, steroids and symptomatic relief.
- **Surgical**: submucosal injection, banding and anal dilatation are used for first- and second-degree haemorrhoids; haemorrhoidectomy is used for third- or fourth-degree haemorrhoids.

2.28 Femoral hernia   Answers: A B C

See also Question 4.20, Paper 4.

A strangulated femoral hernia typically presents as an irreducible lump in the groin, with pain and tenderness. Overlying redness occurs as a result of local inflammation. The hernia may contain omental fat or bowel. If there is obstruction, then vomiting, abdominal distension and constipation occur.

A fluid thrill on coughing suggests a saphena varix.

2.29 Gallstones   Answers: B C D

The following are the modes of presentation of gallstones:

- Asymptomatic, ie an incidental finding
- Acute cholecystitis: this occurs when a stone in the cystic duct or bile duct causes inflammation and transient obstruction
- Chronic cholecystitis
- Biliary colic resulting from attempts to pass the stone
- Acute pancreatitis when stones impact in the ampulla of Vater
- Obstructive jaundice
- Small bowel obstruction caused by 'gallstone ileus'; stones may impact in the terminal ileum
- Empyema: a pus-filled gallbladder after stone impaction causes a swinging pyrexia and systemic illness
- Perforation of the gallbladder, producing peritonitis
- Pain referred to the right shoulder.

2.30 Hydatid disease   Answers: B C D E

Hydatid disease is caused by *Echinococcus granulosus*. It is common in sheep-rearing areas. Humans ingest the ova from the soil on vegetables; the ova pass to the liver via the portal circulation and form cysts within the liver. These may be asymptomatic. The cyst wall may become calcified in which case it is visible on a plain abdominal radiograph.

The clinical features include:

- obstructive jaundice
- malaise
- pruritis
- anaphylaxis.

The cyst may rupture into the following:

- The biliary tree, producing cholangitis or jaundice
- The lung, producing haemoptysis
- The peritoneum, producing peritonitis
- The bowel and hence pass in the faeces.

Failed medical treatment, high risk of rupture or complications are the indications for surgery, when the cyst is excised.

2.31 Swelling at the angle of the jaw   Answers: B D

A pharyngeal pouch is a diverticulum of the pharynx occurring at the junction between the pharynx and the oesophagus. It is the result of incoordination of the inferior constrictor muscle during swallowing, which causes a rise in the pressure within the pharynx. This results in a bulge at a weak point. The typical symptom is regurgitation of undigested food. This may cause hoarseness of the voice. The pouch presses on the oesophagus and causes dysphagia and weight loss. Chest infections may occur if food is aspirated. A swelling is rare but if present it occurs low, behind the sternocleidomastoid muscle. The diagnosis is made on barium swallow. Treatment is by surgical excision.

Enlarged lymph nodes are the most common cause of a lump in the neck. They are the result of infection or neoplasia.

A thyroglossal cyst occurs in the midline, along the thyroglossal tract. It moves on swallowing and on protrusion of the tongue.

A carotid body tumour arises in the chemoreceptor tissue at the carotid bifurcation, level with the hyoid bone. It occurs slightly lower than a branchial cyst. It is deep to the anterior edge of sternocleidomastoid and may be pulsatile. It can be moved from side to side but not up and down. Treatment is by surgical removal.

Thyroid tissue tends to extend retrosternally, not towards the jaw.

2.32 Breast carcinoma   Answers: A D E

Breast carcinoma is the most common carcinoma in women. It commonly occurs in women aged over 40 years and the incidence increases with age. Only 1% of breast cancers occur in men. The aetiology is unknown. However, risk factors include the following:

- Genetic factors: women who have first-degree relatives with breast/ovarian cancer are at increased risk
- Environmental: there is a geographical distribution, eg there is a low incidence in Japan
- Previous breast cancer: when one breast is affected the risk is increased in the other breast
- Nulliparous women and those who had their first pregnancy over the age of 30 years: it is thought that oestrogens unopposed by progesterones increase susceptibility
- Ionising radiation
- Obesity (oestrogens are produced in peripheral fat).

The following are protective factors:

- Early first pregnancy
- Breast-feeding.

The incidence of breast carcinoma does not appear to be affected by the oral contraceptive pill, but is increased by HRT.

2.33 Scrotal swelling   Answers: C D

A hydrocele envelops the testis and the testis is usually not palpable.
An indirect inguinal hernia may extend into the scrotum but does not trans-illuminate.

An encysted hydrocele of the cord in the scrotum is separate from the testis and transilluminates.

An epididymal cyst is fluid filled and separate from the testis. Therefore the testis is palpable separately.

Epididymal tuberculosis causes swelling confined to the scrotum; there is thickening of the cord, which feels hard. It does not transilluminate.

2.34 Acute renal failure   Answers: A B C D

Postoperatively, renal failure develops in the following conditions:

- Lack of renal perfusion, ie hypovolaemia caused by haemorrhage or dehydration
- Infection, especially Gram-negative septicaemia
- In patients who have pre-existing renal disease.

An accurate fluid chart is required to monitor fluid balance. Furosemide (frusemide) or dopamine may be used to promote diuresis. Hyperkalaemia and acidosis occur.

A renal calculus is unlikely to cause acute renal failure postoperatively (because this would have to affect both kidneys), but obstruction of a ureter may result in hydronephrosis and reduced renal function.

2.35 Extradural haemorrhage   Answer: C

The classic history of an extradural haemorrhage is loss of consciousness with a 'lucid interval' before a deterioration in the Glasgow Coma Scale (GCS) score. It is usually caused by damage to the middle meningeal artery. Haematoma develops between the dura and the skull, raising intracranial pressure. The lateralising signs are an ipsilateral dilated pupil and contralateral hemiparesis.

A skull fracture may not be present and there may no history of loss of consciousness.

Raised intracranial pressure causes a rise in blood pressure and a fall in heart rate.

Treatment includes:

- mannitol (an osmotic diuretic)
- evacuation of haematoma via a burr hole or craniotomy.

2.36 Undescended testis   Answers: C D

An undescended testis lies anywhere along the course of descent from the abdomen to the scrotum. It is usually accompanied by a congenital inguinal hernia. Most cases are recognised in infancy or childhood and should be corrected early, if possible by the age of 2 years. An undescended testis predisposes to malignancy. The affected testis may be small and fertility may be impaired, but, if the other testis is functioning normally, this prevents sterility. There is an increased risk of torsion.

2.37 Varicocele   Answers: C D E

A varicocele is a collection of dilated veins of the pampiniform plexus. It is much more common on the left than on the right side. It is associated with renal tumours on the left side because this may obstruct drainage of the left testicular vein into the left renal vein.

The patient complains of a lump and/or an aching dull pain. A varicocele is likened to 'a bag of worms'. It is more noticeable when the patient is standing. It may be associated with infertility. Treatment is conservative but in troublesome cases embolisation can be performed. Alternatively, the veins can be ligated and divided.

2.38 Raynaud's phenomenon   Answers: C E

Raynaud's phenomenon describes certain changes of the hands or feet occurring in response to cold. Classically the fingers first turn white as a result of arterial spasm and the fingers become cold. Then they turn blue as a result of cyanosis and finally they turn red as a result of reactive hyper-aemia; this is painful.

Raynaud's phenomenon may be idiopathic but it is associated with the following:

- A cervical rib
- Cervical spondylosis

- Connective tissue disorders, eg rheumatoid arthritis
- Oesophagitis (note that oesophagitis occurs and not oesophageal carcinoma), CREST syndrome (**c**alcinosis, **R**aynaud's phenomenon, (o)**e**sophageal dysfunction, **s**clerodactyly and **t**elangiectasia), scleroderma and telangiectasia
- Use of vibratory tools
- Arterial disease, eg atherosclerosis and emboli from the subclavian artery
- Drugs, eg α-receptor stimulants
- Blood disorders, eg hyperviscosity.

Do not confuse with Raynaud's disease which is idiopathic.

2.39 Pancreatitis – complications   Answers: C E

The following are the main complications of acute pancreatitis:

- Pseudocyst formation
- Pancreatic abscess
- Acute respiratory distress syndrome (ARDS)
- Pleural effusions
- Renal failure
- Ileus: this is not caused by obstruction
- Shock: hypovolaemia and tachycardia
- Diabetes mellitus
- Metabolic effects: albumin falls, hypocalcaemia, hypomagnesaemia
- Necrotising haemorrhagic pancreatitis: fat necrosis can cause embolism; also calcium is sequestered
- Haemorrhage: into a pseudocyst or due to peptic ulceration.

Carcinoma of the pancreas and stones in the ampulla of Vater cause acute pancreatitis; hyperparathyroidism, hypercalcaemia and hyperlipidaemia predispose to pancreatitis.

2.40 Rodent ulcers   Answer: B

A 'rodent ulcer' is a basal cell carcinoma. It characteristically presents on the upper part of the face and ears, especially on sun-exposed areas, but can occur on the neck or anywhere else on the body. It presents as a pearly white nodule with telangiectasia. As it enlarges, it may ulcerate with a pearly rolled edge.

Basal cell carcinomas do not metastasise. They are malignant by way of their local invasion and can cause significant tissue damage by eroding into local tissue.

Treatment:

- Local excision
- Radiotherapy (very effective)
- Cryotherapy.

2.41 Tetany   Answers: A B D

Tetany is the muscle spasm that occurs in hypocalcaemia.

A metabolic alkalosis raises the pH as the H^+ concentration falls. This causes calcium to move into cells (hence the serum calcium level is reduced) and results in muscle twitching.

In thyroidectomy, a well-known complication is the removal of the parathyroid glands. This results in reduced parathyroid hormone and a fall in serum calcium.

A dirty wound causes tetanus, not tetany!

Overbreathing causes the $P\text{co}_2$ to fall, ie respiratory alkalosis. Hypocalcaemia occurs and the muscles become hyperexcitable.
Hypokalaemia is a recognised cause of paralytic ileus, not hypocalcaemia.

2.42 Ingrowing toenail   Answers: C D E

An ingrowing toenail occurs when the nail grows downwards into the soft tissue adjacent to it. It most commonly occurs on the lateral side of the big toe. It becomes infected and swollen, causing pain and discomfort. The treatment is the following:

- To cut the nail square and keep it clean
- Antibiotics are used in the acute stage for local infection
- Surgical treatment includes wedge excision of the nail and nail bed or avulsion of the nail and nail bed. This is best done after the acute infection has settled, but may be necessary to eliminate infection.

2.43 Upper gastrointestinal (GI) bleed   Answers: D E

Haematemesis of 1 L is a medical emergency. Resuscitation is mandatory, with attention to the airway, breathing and circulation (ABC).

Intravenous access is obtained and fluid loss is replaced with blood, colloid or crystalloid. Blood should be sent for a full blood count (FBC), urea and electrolytes (U&Es), clotting screen and crossmatch. Pulse rate, blood pressure and respiratory rate are monitored. (Hypovolaemia causes low blood pressure and tachycardia.) A central venous pressure line is useful to maintain fluid balance.

Gastroscopy is performed as soon as possible (within 6 hours), particularly in patients aged over 65, in patients who have a postural drop in blood pressure, where there is persistent tachycardia and when haemoglobin is < 10 g/dL.

Gastroscopy is performed to identify the source of the blood loss and facilitates treatment such as injection sclerotherapy. Surgery is indicated in persistent bleeding.

2.44 Pilonidal sinus   Answers: A D E

A pilonidal sinus is a sinus containing hairs. It commonly occurs in hair-bearing areas and may become infected to produce a pilonidal abscess. The most common site is the natal cleft, but it is also seen in the fingers of hair-dressers where hairs become implanted under the skin. A pilonidal sinus tends to persist, with chronic discharge via one or more sinuses to the skin. Treatment is by excision of the sinus with surrounding tissue.

2.45 Malignant melanoma   Answers: A B C

Malignant melanoma is a malignant tumour of melanocytes. It commonly occurs on the soles of the feet and on the head and neck. It can occur in the nail bed, eye or mouth. Malignant melanoma is associated with exposure to ultraviolet light. The highest incidence is seen in Queensland, Australia. The incidence is lower in black populations.

Most tumours are pigmented but some have no pigment, ie they are amelanotic. Changes in the appearance of a mole should arouse suspicion. Malignant melanomas itch, bleed and ulcerate. Some undergo spontaneous regression but this is not associated with hypophysectomy.

The treatment of choice is surgery, with wide excision of the lesion. Radiotherapy and chemotherapy are used for palliation in cases that have spread.

2.46 Carotid artery stenosis   Answers: A B D

Carotid artery occlusion usually occurs at the carotid bifurcation. It often goes unnoticed because the brain receives a contralateral blood supply via the circle of Willis.

Patients present with transient ischaemic attacks causing weakness in the contralateral limbs or amaurosis fugax, which is a transient loss of vision in the ipsilateral eye. These resolve within a few hours. The cause is emboli from the carotid circulation impacting in smaller intracerebral vessels.

Vomiting is not a sign of carotid disease. It would indicate disease of the posterior circulation.

Patients with symptoms and stenosis > 70% should be treated with endarterectomy.

2.47 Compound fracture of a bone   Answers: B C

A compound fracture is also known as an 'open fracture'. It is a fracture of a bone with breach of the overlying skin, allowing access to the exterior. This poses a major risk of infection.

The following is the first-line treatment:

- To cover the wound with an iodine-soaked dressing
- Antibiotic prophylaxis with penicillin and flucloxacillin (or suitable alternative)
- Tetanus immunisation
- Débridement
- Skeletal stabilisation.

Operative fixation may be carried out at this stage.

2.48 H$_2$-receptor antagonists   Answers: A C D

Ranitidine is an H$_2$-receptor antagonist. It acts by blocking the histamine receptors in the stomach, thereby reducing gastric acid secretion. Cimetidine is another example. Both may be given orally or intravenously. In upper GI bleeding, they have been superseded by PPIs such as omeprazole, lansoprazole and pantoprazole. These are also useful in the prevention of stress ulcers when there is risk in major operations and are given pre- and postoperatively.

2.49 Ulcerative colitis versus Crohn's disease   Answers: A D

Feature	Ulcerative colitis	Crohn's disease
Rectal bleeding	+++	+
Diarrhoea	+++	+
Steatorrhoea and malabsorption	–	+ + +
Rectal involvement	+++	+
Abdominal mass	+ –	++
Perianal lesions	+/–	+ + +
Fistulae	+/–	+ + +
Toxic megacolon	++	+/–
Malignant change	++	+/–

2.50 Dupuytren's contracture   Answers: A B

Dupuytren's contracture (or cord) is a contracture of the palmar fascia. The cause is idiopathic but there is a familial component (autosomal dominant inheritance).

A flexor deformity of the finger develops, which may be debilitating. It may occur bilaterally. Cord excision is indicated if it affects daily life.

2.51 Femoral shaft fracture   Answers: A B D

The femur is a large bone and its fracture involves a considerable amount of trauma. Blood loss into the surrounding soft tissue is significant and may result in shock. Intravenous fluid replacement is required.

In closed fractures, fat embolism (from bone marrow) is a common complication.

Tetanus immunisation is mandatory in open fractures.

Internal fixation of the femur is by intramedullary nailing.

Healing of the femur takes at least 3 months.

2.52 Postoperative oliguria   Answers: C D

Urinary retention is a common postoperative complication occurring within 24 hours, especially in men. Examination of the abdomen is appropriate to look for an enlarged bladder. A urinary catheter may then be inserted and is diagnostic as well as therapeutic. Poor urine output may also be caused by hypovolaemia. This is assessed with a fluid challenge of 200 mL, given intravenously, which should raise urine output. If there is no response after rehydration, 40 mg furosemide, a loop diuretic, can be given. However, furosemide can be nephrotoxic and so care must be taken where renal failure is suspected. Persistent hypovolaemia causes acute renal failure. After rehydration, dopamine may be required to stimulate renal function. Mannitol is an osmotic diuretic and would not be appropriate. Haemodialysis is used in the late stages of renal failure.

2.53 Cellulitis   Answer: C

Cellulitis is inflammation of subcutaneous tissue that spreads locally. It is usually caused by S*treptococcus pyogenes*. The area of skin is typically red, hot and tender. Spreading cellulitis requires urgent treatment with antibiotics, (such as intravenous penicillin). Localised infection may lead to a collection of pus in the form of an abscess, which requires incision and drainage. Cellulitis can occur with malignancy and for infection, but is not diagnostic of these.

2.54 Salivary duct calculi   Answers: B C D

The aetiology of salivary duct calculi is unknown. They are more common in the submandibular duct than in the parotid duct. The acute inflammation of the salivary glands occurring in mumps is more common in the parotid gland.

The calculi cause obstruction of the duct and stasis of saliva, which increases the risk of infection. Clinically, the features are the following:

- Painful swelling of the gland, which is usually unilateral
- Pain on eating meals as saliva production increases
- A foul taste in the mouth
- Sudden relief of symptoms.

The standard investigations are plain radiographs and sialography. Submandibular duct calculi tend to be quite large and are therefore calcified. This shows up on a radiograph. Parotid duct calculi, however, tend to be small and are often radiolucent.

An ultrasound scan is useful to diagnose an abscess.

Treatment: sucking a lemon or lemon sweets stimulates salivation, which 'flushes' out the salivary ducts of calculi. Otherwise, open removal is required.

2.55 Carcinoma of the stomach   Answers: B C D E

Carcinoma of the stomach is common. It occurs in men more often than in women, in a ratio of 2:1. It is most common in the antrum. It may occur as a result of malignant transformation of a polyp or as a primary lesion. The symptoms include epigastric pain, loss of appetite, loss of weight, dysphagia, regurgitation and vomiting. The patient appears cachectic. An epigastric mass may be palpable, with tenderness and obstruction. Fluid in the stomach causes a succussion splash. There may be iron deficiency and/or pernicious anaemia. Metastases occur in the following ways:

- By local invasion
- Via the lymphatics:
    - to the liver, causing ascites, hepatomegaly and jaundice
    - to the lungs, causing pleural effusions
    - to the brain
    - to lymph nodes (an enlarged lymph node in the left supraclavicular fossa is called Virchow's node or Troisier's sign)
- Via the bloodstream
- By transcoelomic spread.

Metastases to the ovaries cause Krukenberg's tumours.

Surgical treatment is gastrectomy – total or partial – but the recurrence rate in the remnant is significant.

Prognosis depends on the extent of spread. In general, patients tend to present late and therefore prognosis is poor – a 5-year survival rate of 10–25%.

2.56 Ureteric calculi   Answers: A D

The symptoms of ureteric calculi include loin pain that is colicky or constant, radiating into the groin and scrotum. The patient may roll about in pain with little relief. Microscopic or macroscopic haematuria occurs.

Approximately 70% of stones contain calcium oxalate, 15% are mixed phosphate stones and 8% are uric acid.

'Triple phosphate' stones are composed of calcium, magnesium and ammonium phosphate. This forms the typical 'staghorn calculus'. It is caused by the urease-producing organism *Proteus* species.

Stone formation is increased in the following:

- Hyperparathyroidism (increased calcium)
- Gout
- Cystinuria.

Urinary stasis predisposes to the precipitation of crystals and stone formation.

Infection producing alkaline urine causes the precipitation of calcium.

Schistosomiasis predisposes to bladder calculi.

Treatment of ureteric calculi includes the following:

- Analgesia, eg diclofenac, for symptomatic relief
- Lithotripsy
- Ureteroscopic removal
- Surgery.

Ureteric calculi do not predispose to transitional cell carcinoma of the ureter.

Bladder calculi cause irritation and an increased incidence of bladder tumours of the squamous cell type.

2.57 Metabolic response to trauma   Answers: B C E

Remember that trauma refers to all types of injury, whether accidental or surgical. The physiological response occurs in two phases:

1. The ebb phase: this occurs in the first 24 hours. During this time there is:
    –   increased sympathetic activity
    –   increased acute phase proteins
    –   mobilisation of energy reserves (glucose and triglyceride levels increase)
    –   decreased insulin secretion
    –   increased adrenocorticotrophic hormone (ACTH): this causes a rise in cortisol levels and thus sodium and water retention with – release of ADH to maintain blood pressure by fluid retention
2. The flow phase: this occurs days to weeks later:
    –   metabolic rate is increased
    –   nitrogen excretion is increased as a result of protein catabolism – protein loss occurs from skeletal muscle breakdown, resulting in loss of lean body mass
    –   energy is consumed
    –   insulin resistance occurs.

2.58 Rectal bleeding – bright red   Answers: B E

The passage of bright red blood with the stool is usually a result of local pathology.

Haemorrhoids are a common cause. However, a thrombosed pile consists of solid clot and altered blood, which is dark red. Therefore, fresh red bleeding does not occur.

Anal fissure: constipation causes trauma to the fissure which opens up and causes bleeding.

Neoplasia, eg adenoma or carcinoma of the rectum: these are situated close to the anal margin and can cause fresh red bleeding. More proximal colonic carcinoma would cause blood to be mixed in with the stool.

Trauma: local injury.

Note that the question specifies 'bright red blood' but there are numerous other causes of rectal bleeding (see also Question 3.58, Paper 3).

An ischiorectal abscess occurs in the ischiorectal fossa, the main symptom being pain.

2.59 Staging of breast carcinoma   Answers: A B

Staging of breast tumours is used to assess spread, predict prognosis and facilitate treatment.

Diagnosis is made by:

- ultrasonography
- mammography
- fine-needle aspiration or biopsy
- lumpectomy.

Staging is done using the TNM classification:

T = tumour size and extent (T0–T4, Tis representing 'carcinoma *in situ*')

N = spread to lymph nodes (N0–N3)

M = metastases (M0 or M1, indicating the presence or absence of metastases).

Stage	Features	Five-year survival rate (%)
I	Tumour ≤ 2 cm	85
II	Tumour ≤ 5 cm	
	Nodes not fixed	65
III	Tumour ≤ 5 cm	
	Supraclavicular nodes fixed	40
IV	Distant metastases	10

Treatment: in localised disease, ie for stages I and II, surgery is indicated. This includes wide local excision or mastectomy, axillary clearance and adjuvant radiotherapy and/or chemotherapy and/or endocrine therapy.

If metastases are present, ie stages III and IV, treatment is palliative, with radiotherapy and drugs, eg tamoxifen, corticosteroids and chemotherapy, and newer aromatase inhibitors.

2.60 Hypocalcaemia   Answers: C E

Calcium is present largely in bones; a small amount is present in blood, both as ions and bound to albumin. If acidity [H^+] increases, free calcium ions increase. Calcium levels must be corrected with respect to albumin as follows:

Corrected calcium = [Measured calcium + (40 – Albumin)] × 0.02

Calcium levels depend on intake and loss.

The causes of hypocalcaemia are:

- hypoparathyroidism
- chronic renal failure
- vitamin D deficiency
- septicaemia
- acute pancreatitis (gallstones can cause this but do not cause hypocalcaemia directly).

In thyroidectomy, a complication is removal of the parathyroid glands, which results in hypocalcaemia.

In low calcium states, replacement is with intravenous calcium gluconate.

In multiple myeloma and other malignancy, calcium levels tend to be raised. Parathyroid adenoma causes hypercalcaemia as a result of excess parathyroid hormone secretion.

BEST OF FIVE AND MULTIPLE CHOICE QUESTIONS PAPER 3

60 questions: time allowed 2½ hours

Best of Five Questions
Mark your answers with a tick (True) in the box provided.

3.1   A 55-year-old Asian woman was seen in the surgical outpatient clinic with a chronic ulcer on her left forearm. On enquiry by the consultant she revealed that she suffered a full-thickness burn at the site of the ulcer almost 25 years ago. The consultant told the patient that she had a Marjolin's ulcer. Which of the following statements best describes a Marjolin's ulcer?

- ☐ A   It is a sarcoma that develops in a scar
- ☐ B   It grows rapidly
- ☐ C   It is usually associated with secondary deposits in the regional lymph nodes
- ☐ D   It is painless
- ☐ E   It is the result of localised areas of fat necrosis

3.2   A 45-year-old man who had previously undergone laparotomy for removal of a malignant growth involving the colon presented in the surgical outpatient clinic with a persistent sinus in his midline laparotomy scar. Which of the following conditions is least likely to be associated with persistence of a sinus?

- ☐ A   Presence of a foreign body or necrotic tissue
- ☐ B   Inefficient or non-dependent drainage
- ☐ C   Unrelieved obstruction of the lumen of a viscus
- ☐ D   Irradiation
- ☐ E   Excess vitamin C intake

3.3   A 20-year-old woman of African origin had a benign breast lump
        removed from her right breast. Two months later there is a firm,
        2 × 1.5 cm nodular mass with intact overlying epithelium in the
        region of the incision. On examination the scar is firm, but not
        tender, with no erythema. This mass is excised and
        microscopically shows fibroblasts with abundant collagen. Which
        of the following mechanisms has most probably produced this
        series of events?

❑   A   Development of a fibrosarcoma
❑   B   Keloid formation
❑   C   Poor wound healing
❑   D   Foreign body response from suturing
❑   E   Staphylocccal wound infection

3.4   A 50-year-old man was investigated for vague abdominal
        discomfort of 6 months' duration. His clinical examination was
        negative for lymphadenopathy, abdominal masses or
        organomegaly. Bowel sounds were audible. A stool specimen
        tested for occult blood was negative. Abdominal computed
        tomography (CT) showed a 20 cm retroperitoneal soft tissue mass
        obscuring the left psoas muscle. Which of the following
        neoplasms is this man most likely to have?

❑   A   Melanoma
❑   B   Hamartoma
❑   C   Adenocarcinoma
❑   D   Lymphoma
❑   E   Liposarcoma

3.5   An 85-year-old woman fell from stairs and presented in A&E with
        a painful left hip and an inability to ambulate. Radiographs
        showed not only a fracture of the left femoral head, but also a
        compressed fracture of the T10 vertebra. She was previously fit
        with an unremarkable past medical history. Which of the
        following conditions is she most likely to have?

❑   A   Acute osteomyelitis
❑   B   Osteogenesis imperfecta
❑   C   Osteoporosis
❑   D   Polyostotic fibrous dysplasia
❑   E   Metastatic breast carcinoma

3.6 A 26-year-old woman is diagnosed with a phaeochromocytoma. The urine levels of which of the following substances will be high in this patient?

- ❏ A Metanephrines
- ❏ B Dehydroepiandrosterone
- ❏ C Pregnanetriol
- ❏ D Cortisol
- ❏ E 5-Hydroxyindoleacetic acid

3.7 A 50-year-old man is admitted to the intensive care unit (ICU) after acute haemorrhagic pancreatitis. On day 3 he develops acute respiratory distress syndrome (ARDS). Which of the following variables is most likely to be lower than normal in this patient?

- ❏ A Oncotic pressure of alveolar fluid
- ❏ B Lung compliance
- ❏ C Work of breathing
- ❏ D Alveolar–arterial pressure difference
- ❏ E Surface tension of alveolar fluid

3.8 A jaundiced patient has predominantly conjugated hyperbilirubinaemia. Which of the following conditions is most likely to be associated with conjugated hyperbilirubinaemia?

- ❏ A Haemolysis caused by hereditary spherocytosis
- ❏ B Haemolysis resulting from rhesus incompatibility
- ❏ C Acute haemolytic crisis in sickle cell disease
- ❏ D Obstructive jaundice caused by carcinoma of the head of pancreas
- ❏ E Gilbert syndrome

3.9 A 55-year-old man undergoes abdominoperineal resection for an advanced colorectal carcinoma. His baseline blood pressure is 140/80 mmHg. Intraoperatively there was faecal contamination of the peritoneal cavity. Postoperatively, on return to the ICU, the patient is mechanically ventilated and his blood pressure is 90/50 mmHg. His urinary output is 20 mL in the first hour. Which of the following is the best strategy to improve his urine output?

- A Start infusion of an inotrope
- B Fluid challenge followed by vasopressor
- C Give intravenous corticosteroids
- D Insert a Swan–Ganz catheter
- E Use a stroke-volume monitor

3.10 **A 45-year-old woman with a previous history of multiple gallstones has developed jaundice as a result of a large stone obstructing the common bile duct. Which of the following biochemical abnormalities will be seen in this patient?**

- A Decreased bilirubin in the urine
- B Increased urobilinogen in the urine
- C Decreased urobilinogen in the stool
- D Decreased plasma direct bilirubin
- E Decreased plasma conjugated bilirubin

3.11 **A 12-year-old boy with a history of hay fever and eczema was brought to A&E after being stung by a bee. The attending doctor immediately gave this boy a shot of epinephrine (adrenaline). The epinephrine is injected to prevent:**

- A Local immune complex formation
- B Interleukin release from macrophages
- C Binding of anti-receptor antibody
- D Complement activation
- E Systemic anaphylaxis

3.12 **A 40-year-old man who is a heavy smoker was seen in the surgical outpatient clinic complaining of severe pain in both legs even at rest. On examination he had chronic ulceration of his toes. Which of the following conditions is he most likely to have?**

- A Buerger's disease
- B Wegener's granulomatosis
- C Kawasaki's disease
- D Polyarteritis nodosa
- E Takayasu's arteritis

3.13   **A patient develops a pneumothorax as a result of spontaneous rupture of an apical bulla. In this patient:**

❏   A   The lung expands outwards and the chest wall springs inwards
❏   B   The lung expands outwards and the chest wall springs outwards
❏   C   The lung collapses inwards and the chest wall collapses inwards
❏   D   The lung collapses inwards and the chest wall springs outwards
❏   E   The lung volume is unaffected and chest wall springs outwards

3.14   **A 22-year-old motorcyclist was brought to A&E after a road traffic accident (RTA). On examination he had a large bruise on his right arm with inability to move his arm. A radiograph of the right arm revealed a fracture involving the surgical neck of the humerus. Such a fracture is most likely to injure:**

❏   A   The subscapular artery
❏   B   The circumflex scapular artery
❏   C   The radial recurrent artery
❏   D   The brachial artery
❏   E   The posterior humeral circumflex artery

3.15   **A 45-year-old man presented in A&E with massive haematemesis. An emergency endoscopy was performed, which shows a bleeding gastric ulcer of the lesser curvature of the stomach. The most likely vessel to be involved is:**

❏   A   The left gastroepiploic artery
❏   B   The right gastroepiploic artery
❏   C   The gastroduodenal artery
❏   D   The left gastric artery
❏   E   The short gastric arteries

Multiple Choice Questions

Mark your answers with a tick (True) or a cross (False) in the box provided. Leave the box blank for 'Don't know'. Do not look at the answers until you have completed the whole question paper.

3.16 Colles' fracture:

❑ A Requires manipulation of the humerus with immobilisation for 6 weeks
❑ B May lead to delayed rupture of extensor pollicis longus
❑ C Can be manipulated under local anaesthesia
❑ D Occurs after a fall on to the outstretched hand
❑ E Usually unites in 6 weeks

3.17 Epistaxis:

❑ A Is bleeding from the epiglottis
❑ B Usually occurs from Little's area
❑ C Can cause a drop in blood pressure
❑ D Can be treated with nasal packing
❑ E May require internal carotid artery ligation

3.18 Laparoscopic cholecystectomy:

❑ A Is routinely performed for elective cholecystectomy
❑ B Has the advantage of small incisions, compared with open cholecystectomy
❑ C Has no complications
❑ D Is contraindicated in elderly people
❑ E Is used for appendicitis

3.19 Hypercalcaemia causes:

❑ A Renal stones
❑ B Polyuria
❑ C Constipation
❑ D Gallstones
❑ E Tetanus

3.20   A supracondylar fracture of the humerus may lead to:

☐   A   Injury to the brachial artery
☐   B   Injury to the ulnar nerve
☐   C   Avascular necrosis of the radius
☐   D   Injury of the axillary artery
☐   E   Infarction of the forearm muscles

3.21   Gallstone ileus:

☐   A   Causes large bowel obstruction
☐   B   Causes small bowel obstruction
☐   C   Is caused by lack of contraction of the gallbladder
☐   D   May result in an abdominal radiograph showing gas in the biliary tree
☐   E   Is treated by cholecystostomy

3.22   Blood transfusion:

☐   A   Can cause a reaction that may manifest as pruritis
☐   B   Should be stopped if pyrexia develops
☐   C   Uses blood that has been screened for hepatitis B antibody
☐   D   Reactions are most often a result of blood mismatch
☐   E   Reaction may lead to jaundice

3.23   A swelling with expansile pulsation above the left clavicle may be:

☐   A   Pancoast's tumour
☐   B   An aneurysm of the subclavian artery
☐   C   A dilated subclavian vein
☐   D   Virchow's node
☐   E   A branchial cyst

3.24   Features consistent with a diagnosis of acute ulcerative colitis include:

☐   A   A normal barium enema
☐   B   Tachycardia > 100/min
☐   C   Weight gain
☐   D   Serum albumin < 30 g/L
☐   E   Dilatation of the colon on plain abdominal radiograph

3.25 **Which of the following occur in anterior perforation of peptic ulcers?**

- ❏ A   Board-like rigidity
- ❏ B   An increased area of liver dullness to percussion
- ❏ C   A state of collapse dominating the picture shortly after onset
- ❏ D   Gas under the diaphragm on an erect chest radiograph
- ❏ E   Peritonitis

3.26 **Colonic polyps:**

- ❏ A   May be benign
- ❏ B   May be malignant
- ❏ C   Should be left untreated if asymptomatic
- ❏ D   Of the tubular type in the colon are less likely to undergo malignant change than the villous type
- ❏ E   May occur in Peutz–Jeghers syndrome

3.27 **Crohn's disease:**

- ❏ A   Is associated with finger clubbing
- ❏ B   May cause protein malabsorption
- ❏ C   Is characteristically associated with dilatation of the terminal ileum
- ❏ D   Hardly ever affects the colon
- ❏ E   May undergo spontaneous symptomatic remission

3.28 **A femoral hernia:**

- ❏ A   Should be treated with a truss
- ❏ B   Has the femoral vein lateral to it
- ❏ C   May contain omentum
- ❏ D   Appears above and medial to the inguinal ligament
- ❏ E   Can strangulate the bowel without obstructing it

3.29   In the radiological differentiation between cancer of the colon and diverticulitis, which of the following features would favour a diagnosis of diverticulitis?

❏ A   A long segment of affected bowel
❏ B   An abrupt transition from abnormal to normal bowel
❏ C   Evidence of spasm of the colon
❏ D   Diverticula
❏ E   Apple-core appearance

3.30   Sequelae of acute cholecystitis include:

❏ A   Perforation of the gallbladder
❏ B   Cholecystoduodenal fistula
❏ C   Ascending cholecystitis
❏ D   An enlarged palpable gallbladder
❏ E   Septicaemia

3.31   Ascending cholangitis is associated with:

❏ A   Large bowel obstruction
❏ B   Gallstones
❏ C   Fever
❏ D   Stricture of the common bile duct
❏ E   Cholangiocarcinoma

3.32   Carcinoma of the oesophagus:

❏ A   Is diagnosed at colonoscopy
❏ B   Presents with dysuria
❏ C   Spreads to the liver
❏ D   Can be treated with radiotherapy
❏ E   Can be treated with surgery

3.33   A breast lump that is fixed to skin but not to deep tissues may be:

❏ A   A fibroadenoma
❏ B   A cyst
❏ C   An intraduct papilloma
❏ D   An abscess
❏ E   Fat necrosis

3.34   Clinical findings of a ruptured spleen may include:

❏   A   Haemorrhagic shock
❏   B   Haematemesis
❏   C   Reduced bowel sounds
❏   D   Abdominal distension
❏   E   Shifting dullness within the abdomen

3.35   Predisposing factors in the formation of renal calculi are:

❏   A   Dupuytren's contracture
❏   B   A tropical climate
❏   C   Thyrotoxicosis
❏   D   Parathyroid tumour
❏   E   Malnutrition

3.36   In a case of renal trauma followed by haematuria:

❏   A   The kidney should be explored immediately
❏   B   An intravenous urogram is of no value
❏   C   A CT scan of the abdomen should be obtained
❏   D   Nephrectomy may be required
❏   E   The patient must be followed up

3.37   With regard to ulcerative colitis:

❏   A   Malignancy is a feature
❏   B   Transmural involvement occurs
❏   C   The rectum is always involved
❏   D   It is familial
❏   E   Crypt abscesses are seen

3.38   Recognised complications of venous insufficiency of the lower limb include:

❏   A   Chronic ulceration
❏   B   Superficial phlebitis
❏   C   Stiffness of the ankle joint
❏   D   DVT
❏   E   Localised eczema

3.39   Digital gangrene may be caused by:

☐ A   Frostbite
☐ B   Alcoholism
☐ C   Ergot derivatives
☐ D   Polyneuritis
☐ E   Cervical rib

3.40   An anal fissure:

☐ A   Is associated with a sentinel pile
☐ B   Most commonly lies anteriorly
☐ C   Is an ulcer of the rectal mucosa
☐ D   Is a cause of bleeding in infancy
☐ E   Is a recognised complication of Crohn's disease

3.41   The effect of an arterial embolus depends on:

☐ A   Collateral circulation of the area where the embolus lodges
☐ B   Site of origin
☐ C   Size of the embolus
☐ D   Composition of the embolus
☐ E   Time of onset of thrombolysis

3.42   Coronary artery grafting for ischaemic heart disease:

☐ A   Always requires cardiopulmonary bypass
☐ B   Is usually performed using intercostal arteries as grafts
☐ C   Is unlikely to be successful if more than two major coronary
         arteries are narrowed
☐ D   Requires preceding coronary angiography
☐ E   Has not been shown to prolong life

**3.43   The following are proved methods of prophylaxis in reducing the
         incidence of DVT:**

☐ A   Pneumatic calf compression during operations
☐ B   Subcutaneous low-molecular-weight heparin daily
☐ C   Elasticated compression stockings
☐ D   Aspirin 300 mg four times a day
☐ E   Immobilisation

3.44   Surgical emphysema may be caused by:

- ❏   A   Spontaneous pneumothorax
- ❏   B   Perforation of the oesophagus
- ❏   C   Hyperventilation
- ❏   D   Traumatic pneumothorax
- ❏   E   Smoking

3.45   Anal pain occurs in:

- ❏   A   Carcinoma of the anal canal
- ❏   B   First-degree haemorrhoids
- ❏   C   Anal fissure
- ❏   D   Anal warts
- ❏   E   Perianal haematoma

3.46   The following apply to malignant melanomas:

- ❏   A   They always arise from a pre-existing mole
- ❏   B   The prognosis depends on the depth of invasion
- ❏   C   The prognosis is worse in the superficial spreading form than in the nodular form
- ❏   D   The prognosis is worse in amelanotic lesions
- ❏   E   They metastasise to regional lymph nodes

3.47   The following are features of peripheral arterial disease:

- ❏   A   Intermittent claudication
- ❏   B   Transient ischaemic attacks
- ❏   C   Diabetes mellitus
- ❏   D   Rest pain
- ❏   E   Critical ischaemia

3.48   Infection with tuberculosis (TB) produces:

- ❏   A   A hot red abscess
- ❏   B   Granuloma formation
- ❏   C   Collapse of vertebral bodies
- ❏   D   Epididymitis
- ❏   E   Frequency of micturition

3.49   Carcinoma of the tongue:

☐ A   Is associated with constipation
☐ B   Usually occurs on the posterior third
☐ C   Is associated with the presence of leukoplakia
☐ D   Is usually an adenocarcinoma
☐ E   May be treated by radiotherapy

3.50   A prolapsed lumbar intervertebral disc:

☐ A   Presents with arm pain
☐ B   May cause urinary retention
☐ C   At the level of L3–4 may result in an absent knee jerk
☐ D   May present with buttock pain
☐ E   May be treated conservatively

3.51   Metastases in bone are a common feature of carcinoma of:

☐ A   The kidneys
☐ B   The rectum
☐ C   The lungs
☐ D   The stomach
☐ E   The thyroid

3.52   With regard to an intertrochanteric fracture of the femur:

☐ A   It is common in young men
☐ B   The leg is shortened and externally rotated
☐ C   It is treated with internal fixation
☐ D   There is a high risk of avascular necrosis of the head of the femur
☐ E   It should be treated with total hip replacement

3.53   Concerning antibiotics:

☐ A   A cephalosporin is used prophylactically in cholecystectomy
☐ B   A complete course should be given for prophylaxis in surgery
☐ C   They are the treatment of choice for an abscess
☐ D   Prophylaxis is advised for surgery in patients with prosthetic heart valves
☐ E   Prophylaxis is recommended in colorectal surgery

3.54 Which of the following are complications of urinary catheterisation?

- ☐ A Renal stones
- ☐ B Chronic pyelonephritis
- ☐ C Septicaemia
- ☐ D Prostatitis
- ☐ E Urethral bleeding

3.55 Before starting an urgent operation for large bowel obstruction, which of the following investigations should be carried out?

- ☐ A Full blood count
- ☐ B Chest radiograph
- ☐ C Barium enema
- ☐ D Sigmoidoscopy
- ☐ E Electrolyte concentrations in serum

3.56 In the first 12 hours after a major abdominal operation, particular attention should be paid to:

- ☐ A Urinary output
- ☐ B Pupil size
- ☐ C Wound drainage
- ☐ D Respiration
- ☐ E Core temperature

3.57 Total parenteral nutrition (TPN):

- ☐ A Is beneficial for most malnourished patients preoperatively
- ☐ B Is beneficial for malnourished patients postoperatively
- ☐ C Is usually given via a peripheral intravenous line
- ☐ D Carries a risk of sepsis
- ☐ E Can be given via a nasogastric tube

3.58 Blood may be found on the glove after rectal examination in:

- ☐ A Diverticulitis
- ☐ B Meckel's diverticulum
- ☐ C Carcinoma of the oesophagus
- ☐ D Intussusception
- ☐ E Chronic prostatitis

3.59   **The causes of stricture of the bowel include:**

☐   A   Gluten enteropathy
☐   B   Slow-release potassium tablets
☐   C   Mesenteric ischaemia
☐   D   Crohn's disease
☐   E   Peutz–Jeghers syndrome

3.60   **Volvulus:**

☐   A   Causes venous infarction of the bowel
☐   B   Causes peritonitis
☐   C   Can be cured by performing a barium enema
☐   D   Occurs only in the sigmoid colon
☐   E   Commonly occurs in children and young adults

———————————— **END** ————————————

**Go over your answers until your time is up. Correct answers
and teaching notes are overleaf.**

BEST OF FIVE AND MULTIPLE CHOICE QUESTIONS PAPER 3
Answers

The correct answer options for each question are given below.

3.1	D		3.31	B C D E
3.2	E		3.32	C D E
3.3	B		3.33	D E
3.4	E		3.34	A C D E
3.5	C		3.35	B D E
3.6	A		3.36	C D E
3.7	B		3.37	A C E
3.8	D		3.38	A B C E
3.9	B		3.39	A C E
3.10	C		3.40	A D E
3.11	E		3.41	A C D E
3.12	A		3.42	D
3.13	D		3.43	A B C
3.14	E		3.44	B D
3.15	E		3.45	A C E
3.16	B C D E		3.46	B D E
3.17	B C D		3.47	A B D E
3.18	A B		3.48	B C D E
3.19	A B C		3.49	C E
3.20	A E		3.50	B C D E
3.21	B D		3.51	A C E
3.22	A E		3.52	B C
3.23	B		3.53	A D E
3.24	B D E		3.54	C D E
3.25	A C D E		3.55	A B E
3.26	A B D		3.56	A C D E
3.27	A B E		3.57	B D
3.28	B C E		3.58	A B D
3.29	A C D		3.59	B C D
3.30	A B D E		3.60	A B C

BEST OF FIVE AND MULTIPLE CHOICE QUESTIONS PAPER 3
Answers and Teaching Notes

3.1   D: It is painless

Marjolin's ulcer is carcinoma that develops in a scar. Chronic wounds and scar tissues are prone to an increased risk of skin cancer. In 1828 Jean-Nicholas Marjolin described the occurrence of tumours in post-traumatic scar tissue. Marjolin's ulcer most frequently occurs in old burn scars, but it has also been reported in relation to osteomyelitis, frostbite, venous stasis ulcers, skin graft donor sites, chronic decubitus ulcers, gunshot wounds, puncture wounds, dog bites, occult trauma, injection sites and scar tissue around colostomies. In adults the usual time for the appearance of carcinoma in scar tissue is around 53–59 years of age. As a general rule, the latency period between the burn injury and the appearance of cancer is 25–40 years. It grows slowly, because the scar is relatively avascular, and it is painless because the tissue contains no nerves. Secondary deposits do not occur in the regional lymph nodes because lymphatic vessels have been destroyed. If the ulcer invades normal tissue surrounding the scar, it extends at a normal rate, and lymph nodes are then liable to be involved.

3.2   E: Excess vitamin C intake

Persistence of a sinus or fistula is the result of one of the following:

- A foreign body or necrotic tissue is present, eg a suture, hairs, a sequestrum, a faecolith or even a worm (as in guinea-worm infestation)
- Inefficient or non-dependent drainage: a long, narrow, tortuous track predisposes to inefficient drainage
- Unrelieved obstruction of the lumen of a viscus or tube distal to the fistula
- Absence of rest, such as occurs in fistula *in ano* due to the normal contractions of the sphincter, which also forces faecal matter into the internal opening

- The walls have become lined with epithelium or endothelium (arteriovenous fistula)
- Dense fibrosis prevents contraction and healing
- Type of infection, eg TB or actinomycosis
- The presence of malignant disease
- Persistent discharge, such as urine, faeces or cerebrospinal fluid (CSF)
- Ischaemia
- Drugs, eg steroids
- Malnutrition
- Interference, eg artefacts
- Irradiation, eg rectovaginal fistula after treatment for a carcinoma of the cervix.

3.3   B: Keloid formation

Some individuals have an inappropriate wound-healing response with excessive collagenisation. Excessive formation of the components of the repair process can also complicate wound healing. Aberrations of growth may occur even in what may begin initially as normal wound healing. The accumulation of excessive amounts of collagen may give rise to a raised scar known as a hypertrophic scar; if the scar tissue grows beyond the boundaries of the original wound and does not regress, it is called a keloid. Keloid formation appears to be an individual predisposition, and for unknown reasons this aberration is somewhat more common in African–Americans. The mechanisms of keloid formation are still unknown. Another deviation in wound healing is the formation of excessive amounts of granulation tissue, which protrudes above the level of the surrounding skin and blocks re-epithelialisation. This has been called exuberant granulation (or, with more literary fervour, proud flesh). Excessive granulation must be removed by cautery or surgical excision to permit restoration of the continuity of the epithelium.

Finally (fortunately rarely), incisional scars or traumatic injuries may be followed by exuberant proliferation of fibroblasts and other connective tissue elements, which may, in fact, recur after excision. Called desmoids, or aggressive fibromatoses, these lie in the interface between benign proliferations and malignant (though low-grade) tumours.

The wound will not have excessive collagen with poor wound healing. Sutures can produce small foreign body granulomas, which are typically not visible. Trauma does not lead to neoplasia, so fibrosarcoma is least likely to be seen in this case. A wound infection will produce dehiscence and abscess formation that delays or disrupts collagenisation.

3.4   E: Liposarcoma

Liposarcomas are one of the most common sarcomas of adulthood and appear in adults in their 40s to 60s; they are uncommon in children. They usually arise in the deep soft tissues of the proximal extremities and retroperitoneum, and are notorious for developing into large tumours. Histologically, liposarcomas can be divided into well-differentiated, myxoid, round cell and pleomorphic variants. The well-differentiated variant is relatively indolent, the myxoid type is intermediate in its malignant behaviour, and the round cell and pleomorphic variants are usually aggressive and frequently metastasise. All types of liposarcoma recur locally and often repeatedly unless adequately excised.

Melanomas arise on the skin in most cases and are rarely visceral or in soft tissue. A hamartoma is a peculiar small benign neoplasm composed of tissues normal to a site, but just in a jumbled mass. A pulmonary hamartoma is the most common of these. Adenocarcinomas do not arise in soft tissues. Sarcomas arise in soft tissues. Finally, it is unlikely that matted nodes with lymphoma would reach this size.

3.5   C: Osteoporosis

She most probably has osteoporosis with accelerated bone loss, leading to the propensity for fractures. Physical inactivity further accelerates bone loss and decreases muscle mass and agility, which contribute to falls. Osteoporosis is a disease characterised by increased porosity of the skeleton resulting from reduced bone mass. The associated structural changes predispose the bone to fracture. The disorder may be localised to a certain bone or region, as in disuse osteoporosis of a limb, or may involve the entire skeleton, as a manifestation of a metabolic bone disease. Generalised osteoporosis may be primary, or secondary to a large variety of conditions. The most common forms of osteoporosis are senile and postmenopausal osteoporosis. In these disorders, the critical loss of bone mass makes the skeleton vulnerable to fractures.

An osteomyelitis is not typical at this age and does not usually present as fractures in multiple locations. Osteogenesis imperfecta, an inherited disorder of collagen synthesis, is initially diagnosed in fetuses and young children. Polyostotic fibrous dysplasia is a rare disorder that can be seen with McCune–Albright syndrome. So-called 'pathological fracture' from weakening of bone by metastases can occur, but such patients are often very ill, with a history of weight loss and prior bone pain.

3.6   A: Metanephrines

Phaeochromocytomas are tumours that arise in the adrenal medulla and secrete catecholamines. The principal urinary metabolic products of epinephrine (adrenaline) and norepinephrine (noradrenaline) are the metanephrines, vanillylmandelic acid (VMA) and homovanillic acid (HVA). Normal individuals excrete only very small amounts of these substances in the urine. Normal values for 24 h are as follows: free epinephrine and norepinephrine < 100 μg (< 582 nmol), total metanephrine < 1.3 mg (< 7.1 μmol), VMA < 10 mg (< 50 μmol), and HVA < 15 mg (< 82.4 μmol). In phaeochromocytoma and neuroblastoma, urinary excretion of epinephrine and norepinephrine, and of their metabolic products, increases intermittently. However, excretion of these compounds may also be elevated in: coma, dehydration or extreme stress states; in patients being treated with rauwolfia alkaloids, methyldopa or catecholamines; or after ingestion of foods containing large quantities of vanilla, especially if renal insufficiency is present. All of these compounds may be measured in the same urine specimen.

Urinary dehydroepiandrosterone and pregnanetriol excretion is often increased in congenital adrenal hyperplasia. Free urinary cortisol levels are elevated in Cushing syndrome. Increased urinary excretion of the serotonin metabolite 5-hydroxyindoleacetic acid is seen in functioning carcinoids.

3.7   B: Lung compliance

The development of ARDS starts with damage to the alveolar epithelium and vascular endothelium, resulting in increased permeability to plasma and inflammatory cells, allowing them into the interstitium and alveolar space and resulting in lung oedema. Damage to the surfactant-producing type II cells and the presence of protein-rich fluid in the alveolar space disrupt the production and function of pulmonary surfactant, leading to microatelectasis and impaired gas exchange.

The pathophysiological consequences of lung oedema in ARDS include a decrease in lung volumes, compliance and large intrapulmonary shunts (blood perfusing unventilated segments of the lung). A fall in the residual volume is uniformly present and contributes to ventilation–perfusion inequality. It has been hypothesised that a defective surfactant may be partially responsible for the small lung volumes and that it may worsen oedema accumulation in ARDS (as increases in alveolar surface tension have been shown to increase lung water content by lowering interstitial hydrostatic pressure and increasing interstitial oncotic pressure). The decrease in lung compliance is secondary to the increased lung recoil pressure of the oedematous lung, which clinically increases the work of breathing and leads to respiratory muscle fatigue.

3.8   D: Obstructive jaundice caused by carcinoma of head of pancreas

Bilirubin is a tetrapyrrole created by the normal breakdown of haem. Most bilirubin is produced during the breakdown of haemoglobin and other haemoproteins. Accumulation of bilirubin or its conjugates in body tissues produces jaundice, which is characterised by high plasma bilirubin levels and deposition of yellow bilirubin pigments in skin, sclerae, mucous membranes and other less visible tissues. As bilirubin is highly insoluble in water, it must be converted into a soluble conjugate before elimination from the body. In the liver, uridine diphosphate (UDP)-glucuronyl transferase converts bilirubin to a mixture of monoglucuronides and diglucuronides, referred to as conjugated (direct) bilirubin, which are then secreted into the bile by an ATP-dependent transporter. This process is highly efficient under normal conditions, so plasma unconjugated bilirubin concentrations remain low.

Normal serum values of total bilirubin typically are 0.2–1.0 mg/dL (3.4–17.1 mmol/L), of which no more than 0.2 mg/dL (3.4 mmol/L) reacts directly. Conjugated hyperbilirubinaemia results either from reduced secretion of conjugated bilirubin into the bile, such as occurs in patients with hepatitis, or from impaired flow of bile into the intestine, such as occurs in patients with biliary obstruction as a result of tumours in the head of pancreas. Bile formation is very sensitive to a variety of hepatic insults, including high levels of inflammatory cytokines, such as may occur in patients with septic shock. Diseases that increase the rate of bilirubin formation, such as haemolysis, or diseases that reduce the rate of bilirubin conjugation, such as Gilbert syndrome, produce unconjugated hyperbilirubinaemia.

3.9   B: Fluid challenge followed by vasopressor

Oliguria is hypotension or hypovolaemia until otherwise proven. This patient is likely to be hypovolaemic as well as vasoplegic, secondary to fluid loss in the abdomen and release of inflammatory mediators (particularly inducible nitric oxide synthase) as a result of faecal soiling. The best strategy will be to give him a fluid challenge with 200–250 mL colloid solution followed by infusion of norepinephrine, which is a vasopressor. Unless the low urinary output is caused by poor cardiac performance, there is little to be learned by insertion of a Swan–Ganz catheter. If there is concern that this patient had a history of coronary arterial disease, and may have had a peri-operative myocardial event, a stroke volume monitor may be useful. Inotrope may be indicated if the patient has poor ventricular function. Corticosteroids have no role in this clinical scenario.

3.10 C: Decreased urobilinogen in the stool

Obstruction of intrahepatic or extrahepatic bile ducts prevents the normal delivery of conjugated bilirubin to the duodenum. Hence, conjugated bilirubin (direct bilirubin) regurgitates into the blood, producing jaundice. Conjugated bilirubin is more water soluble than free bilirubin and can be filtered by the kidney and excreted in urine. Intestinal bilirubin is usually metabolised by bacteria in the distal small intestine to produce urobilinogen, a portion of which is reabsorbed into the enterohepatic circulation and can be excreted in the urine. Most of the urobilinogen is further metabolised by colonic bacteria to produce stercobilin, which gives the stool its brown colour. In cases of biliary tree obstruction, bilirubin secretion into the duodenum is reduced and, hence, urinary excretion of urobilinogen is decreased and the presence of urobilinogen and stercobilin in the colon reduced (clay-coloured stools).

3.11 E: Systemic anaphylaxis

Exposure to the allergens of a bee sting is a cause for systemic anaphylaxis for some people. Bee sting will precipitate a type I hypersensitivity reaction and epinephrine can be life saving in this situation.

Local immune complexes are a feature of type III hypersensitivity with farmer's lung. Macrophages have a major role with type IV hypersensitivity reactions. Myasthenia gravis is an example of an anti-receptor disease of an autoimmune nature (type II hypersensitivity). Antibody is directed against acetylcholine receptors. Many myasthenia gravis patients have a thymoma or thymic hyperplasia. Complement activation is a feature of type III hypersensitivity reactions.

3.12 A: Buerger's disease

This patient has Buerger's disease, also known as thromboangiitis obliterans. It is a distinctive disease that often leads to vascular insufficiency. It is characterised by segmental, thrombosing, acute and chronic inflammation of medium-sized and small arteries, principally the tibial and radial arteries, and sometimes secondarily extending to veins and nerves of the extremities.

Previously a condition that occurred almost exclusively among heavy cigarette-smoking men, Buerger's disease has been increasingly reported in women, probably reflecting smoking increases. The disease begins before age 35 in most cases. Later complications are chronic ulceration of the toes, feet or fingers, and frank gangrene in some patients. In contrast to atherosclerosis, Buerger's disease involves smaller arteries and is accompanied by severe pain, even at rest, related undoubtedly to the neural involvement. Abstinence from cigarette smoking in the early stages of the disease often prevents further attacks.

All other conditions are systemic vasculitis of immunological or granulomatous origin.

3.13 D: The lung collapses inwards and the chest wall springs outwards

Pneumothorax is the presence of air within the pleural space. It is considered to be one of the most common forms of thoracic disease and is classified as spontaneous (not caused by trauma), traumatic or iatrogenic. Entry of air into the pleural space results in collapse of the lung. The primary physical sign of pneumothorax is a decrease or absence of breath sounds despite normal or increased resonance on percussion. However, this may be difficult to detect, particularly in patients with a small pneumothorax or in those who have underlying emphysema. Patients with a small pneumothorax (involving < 15% of the hemithorax) may have a normal physical examination. Tachycardia is the most common physical finding.

A large pneumothorax can cause decreased movement of the chest wall, a hyperresonant percussion note, diminished tactile focal fremitus and resonance, and decreased or absent breath sounds on the affected side. Haemodynamic instability, which is indicated by tachycardia, hypotension and cyanosis, suggests a tension pneumothorax. Arterial blood gases may reveal acute respiratory alkalosis and an increased alveolar–arterial oxygen gradient. Unusual clinical manifestations of pneumothorax include ptosis (as a result of extension of subcutaneous emphysema), pneumocephalus (secondary to tension pneumothorax associated with a comminuted fracture of the thoracic spine) and recurrent pneumopericardium (in association with pleuropericardial defect).

3.14 E: Posterior humeral circumflex artery

The posterior and anterior circumflex arteries wrap around the humerus near its surgical neck. A fracture to the surgical neck could damage either of these arteries or the axillary nerve.

The subscapular artery is a branch of the third part of the axillary artery – it branches to form the thoracodorsal artery and the circumflex scapular artery. The radial recurrent artery is a branch of the radial collateral artery – it contributes to collateral circulation around the elbow. The brachial artery is an artery situated deep in the arm – it is close to the humerus, so fracture of the shaft of the humerus at mid-arm might result in damage to this vessel.

3.15 E: Short gastric arteries

The left gastric artery is the artery that supplies the lesser curvature of the stomach (along with the right gastric artery.) These two arteries would be most likely to cause bleeding at the lesser curvature of the stomach. The left gastric is one of the three arteries that comes off the coeliac trunk.

The left and right gastroepiploic arteries are the two arteries that supply the greater curvature of the stomach. The gastroduodenal artery is a branch off the common hepatic artery, which supplies the duodenum, head of pancreas and greater curvature of the stomach. The short gastric arteries are four or five small arteries from the splenic artery which supply the fundus of the stomach.

3.16 Colles' fracture   Answers: B C D E

Colles' fracture is a transverse fracture of the distal radius (± ulna) resulting in a 'dinner-fork' deformity of the wrist. Displacement of the distal fragment requires treatment with manipulation of the wrist under anaesthesia, to align the radius (and ulna if involved).

Extensor pollicis longus may undergo delayed rupture, possibly as a result of damage over the edge of the fractured radius.

Local anaesthesia can be used for a haematoma block or regional block, facilitating manipulation. A fall onto the outstretched hand is the classic history for Colles' fracture, and commonly occurs in elderly women who have osteoporosis.

A plaster is applied to immobilise the distal radius and ulna while the fracture unites over about 6 weeks.

3.17 Epistaxis   Answers: B C D

Epistaxis is bleeding from the nose. The most common site of bleeding is Little's area in the anterior part of the nasal septum. The causes include nose blowing/picking, hypertension, trauma, blood disorders and neoplasia. Continuous bleeding can cause a drop in blood pressure with tachycardia. Appropriate resuscitation is required and the bleeding must be controlled.

Treatment of epistaxis includes the following:

- Nasal packing
- Blood pressure control: hypertension can cause small blood vessels to rupture and therefore requires control
- Cauterisation
- Balloon catheter tamponade
- Vascular ligation in life-threatening cases (of a branch of the external carotid artery).

3.18 Laparoscopic cholecystectomy   Answers: A B

Acute cholecystitis is treated with antibiotics and analgesia. Laparoscopic cholecystectomy can be performed in the acute stage or electively, usually 6 weeks after the acute episode has settled.

The main advantage is the small wound, resulting in an early return to daily activity. The hospital stay is shorter.

Every operation has potential complications. These should be considered as general and specific. The following are the complications related to laparoscopic cholecystectomy:

- Operative:
  - bowel injuries
  - vascular damage/bleeding
  - tension pneumothorax
  - biliary tract injury
  - gallstone spillage
- Postoperative:
  - bleeding
  - biliary leak
  - retained stones
  - pain
- Late: incisional hernia.

The absolute contraindication is bleeding diathesis. The relative contraindications are:

- obesity
- pregnancy
- severe cardiac morbidity
- previous abdominal surgery.

Age is not a contraindication. In fact laparoscopic surgery can be very useful in elderly people.

Laparoscopic cholecystectomy is obviously not used for appendicitis. Appendicectomies are increasingly being performed laparoscopically.

3.19 Hypercalcaemia   Answers: A B C

Hypercalcaemia produces the following:

- Polyuria
- Polydipsia
- Fatigue
- Constipation
- Bone pain
- Urinary tract stones
- Abdominal pain
- Pancreatitis.

Confusion and coma may also occur.

Excess calcium is excreted by the kidneys and therefore leads to the formation of renal stones. In hyperparathyroidism, parathyroid hormone causes reduced calcium excretion and increased phosphate excretion. The phosphate precipitates as calcium salts and paradoxically forms renal stones.

Gallstones are formed mainly of cholesterol and/or bile, with calcium salts being a feature of both.

Constipation is a sign of both hypo- and hypercalcaemia. A fall in plasma calcium increases neuromuscular excitability, causing cramps and tetany. Paraesthesiae occur, especially of the face. Clinically, tapping over the parotid gland causes twitching – Chvostek's sign – and inflating a sphygmomanometer cuff on the arm causes carpal spasm – Trousseau's sign.

Hypocalcaemia occurs in pancreatitis and postoperatively in thyroidectomy patients if the parathyroid glands are affected.

3.20 A supracondylar fracture of the humerus   Answers: A E

Supracondylar fractures are most commonly seen in children. The humerus breaks just above the condyles and the broken edge damages the soft tissues, particularly the brachial artery and median nerve. The brachial artery may go into severe spasm or become kinked. Injury of the brachial artery results in peripheral ischaemia.

The radius receives its blood supply from collateral vessels. Median nerve damage results in loss of abduction of the thumb and loss of sensation over the thumb and lateral two and a half fingers. Median nerve injury tends to recover over a few weeks.

The axillary artery lies in the axilla and is not affected by low humeral damage.

Forearm oedema leads to 'compartment syndrome' which in turn leads to necrosis of the forearm muscles. Fasciotomy is required urgently.

Treatment options for supracondylar fracture are the following:

- Immobilisation in a sling
- Closed reduction under general anaesthesia (GA)
- Open reduction and fixation under GA.

Complications are:

- malunion
- non-union
- stiffness
- myositis ossificans.

3.21 Gallstone ileus   Answers: B D

A complication of gallstones is inflammation of the gallbladder and ulceration into the adjacent duodenum. A cholecystoduodenal fistula results. Stones pass into the duodenum. Gas escapes into the biliary tree and this can be seen on an abdominal radiograph.

A large stone passing into the duodenum can obstruct at the ileocaecal junction, especially when there is a competent ileocaecal valve, causing small bowel obstruction – this is gallstone ileus. Dilated small bowel is seen on an abdominal radiograph. Symptoms include colicky abdominal pain.

The large bowel has a larger calibre; passage of large stones is restricted by the ileocaecal valve. The large bowel therefore does not usually become obstructed.

Treatment is by laparotomy and enterotomy to remove the obstructing stone. The cholecystoduodenal fistula is left *in situ*. Cholecystotomy is not required.

3.22 Blood transfusion   Answers: A E

Complications of blood transfusion include the following:

- Febrile reaction: this is a result of release of pyrogens from cells and immune incompatibility. Pyrexia is a common occurrence and does not necessitate stopping the transfusion. However, if severe (> 38°C), transfusion should be stopped

- Infections transmitted by transfused blood include:
  - viral: with hepatitis A, B, C and D (hepatitis B is screened by identification of the hepatitis B surface antigen, but the problem with this is that it may be absent early after infection); HIV (human immunodeficiency virus), HTLV (human T-lymphotrophic virus), CMV (cytomegalovirus) and EBV (Epstein–Barr virus)
  - bacterial, eg syphilis
  - other, eg malaria.
- Allergic reactions manifest as pruritis, fever, rashes and angio-oedema.
- Haemolytic reactions: haemolysis occurs in major ABO incompatibility, which is usually the result of human error. Features are pyrexia, shortness of breath, loin pain, hypotension, acute renal failure, jaundice and disseminated intravascular coagulation (DIC).

3.23 A swelling with expansile pulsation above the left clavicle   Answer: B

The key descriptions here are 'expansile pulsation' and the site, ie above the clavicle. Pancoast's tumour is a tumour of the lung occurring at the apex of the lung. The site is correct but the tumour would not have pulsation.

The subclavian artery lies between the first rib and the clavicle. It can be tortuous or aneurysmal and this would cause it to be felt above the clavicle.

A cervical rib would exert pressure upwards, causing compression and narrowing. This results in stenosis: the symptoms include upper limb claudication on working with the arm above the head. The segment of artery beyond the stenosis becomes dilated (post-stenotic dilatation) and may form a thrombosis, which may embolise and cause acute ischaemia.

The subclavian vein is not pulsatile.

Virchow's node is a painless enlarged lymph node in the left supraclavicular fossa, suggestive of gastric carcinoma. Palpation of a malignant node at this site is called 'Trosier's sign'.

A branchial cyst is a painless swelling in the side of the neck. The lump lies deep to the sternocleidomastoid muscle at the junction of its upper third and lower two-thirds. It presents in the anterior triangle of the neck. It is not pulsatile.

3.24 Ulcerative colitis

Answers: B D E

Ulcerative colitis presents with recurrent exacerbations of colonic inflammation. This causes diarrhoea, rectal bleeding and abdominal pain. It may lead to dehydration, fever, hypotension and tachycardia. Dilatation of the bowel may result in toxic megacolon and this may eventually perforate and cause peritonitis. Weight loss is common. Profuse diarrhoea with blood loss causes a fall in albumin. (See also Question 1.25, Paper 1; Question 2.49, Paper 2.)

3.25 Perforated peptic ulcer

Answers: A C D E

Perforation of a peptic ulcer is more commonly anterior than posterior. Duodenal ulcer perforation is more common than gastric ulcer perforation. There may be a history of non-steroidal anti-inflammatory drug (NSAID) ingestion.

An erect chest radiograph shows gas under the diaphragm and this is detected clinically by resonance to percussion over the liver. It can be confirmed with a contrast study.

The typical presentation is of sudden-onset epigastric pain with vomiting.

There is rebound tenderness, guarding, board-like rigidity and cardiovascular collapse.

Posterior perforations tend to occur into the lesser sac, which causes the peritonitis to remain localised.

3.26 Colonic polyps

Answers: A B D

A polyp is an abnormal growth of epithelium. It may be pedunculated (on a stalk) or sessile (broad based and flat).

Adenoma describes a benign growth that appears tubular, villous or tubulovillous. In the large bowel all types are pre-malignant. The villous type has the greatest potential for malignant change and is usually sessile, whereas the tubular type has the least potential for malignant change and can be sessile or pedunculated. (The tubulovillous type lies in between.)

Peutz–Jeghers syndrome is an autosomal dominant inherited condition. Numerous polyps occur in the small bowel. These are hamartomas and not adenomas. Spots of brown pigmentation may occur on the lips.

3.27 Crohn's disease   Answers: A B E

Crohn's disease and ulcerative colitis are inflammatory bowel diseases. Both are associated with clubbing. Crohn's disease that affects the small bowel may result in malabsorption of the following:

- Iron (iron deficiency anaemia): absorbed in the duodenum
- Vitamin B$_{12}$ (pernicious anaemia): absorbed in the ileum
- Folate: absorbed in the jejunum
- Protein (malnutrition)
- Fat (steatorrhoea)
- Bile salts (gallstone formation): absorbed in the terminal ileum
- Fat-soluble vitamins, ie vitamins A, D, E and K.

Crohn's disease commonly affects the terminal ileum, producing a 'terminal ileitis'. Inflammation results in narrowing. It affects the colon in about 25% of cases. It also affects the perianal region. The natural history is of chronic inflammatory disease with periods of relapse and remission.

3.28 Femoral hernia   Answers: B C E

Although a truss may be useful, elective surgery for a femoral hernia is advised. It should be arranged at the earliest opportunity because femoral hernias have a high risk of strangulation. In patients who have high-risk co-morbidity, a truss is used to prevent strangulation.

Femoral hernias may contain omentum, fat, lymph nodes or bowel.

The anatomy is: femoral nerve, artery, vein and femoral canal, from lateral to medial. (Aide memoire NAVY)

A femoral hernia appears below the inguinal ligament and lateral to the pubic tubercle.

As with any bowel hernia, it can strangulate without obstruction (see Question 4.20, Paper 4). The bowel can be kinked, trapping one side of the bowel wall but not the entire lumen – Richter's hernia.

3.29 Radiological features of carcinoma of the colon
versus diverticular disease   Answers: A C D

Read the question carefully. It is easy to confuse the diagnoses.

On a barium enema, carcinoma of the colon presents as an apple-core stricture, with shouldering. Obstruction results in dilatation proximal to the stricture.

In contrast, diverticular disease is seen as numerous pockets – a saw-tooth appearance, which is caused by numerous diverticula. A stricture in this case tends to affect a long segment of bowel and there may be spasm. Obstruction can also occur.

In both conditions, an abscess may appear as a gas bubble and, if perforation occurs, there may be gas under the diaphragm.

3.30 Acute cholecystitis   Answers: A B D E

Inflammation of the gallbladder may spread along the cystic and bile ducts towards the liver, causing ascending cholangitis, not cholecystitis (read the question carefully!). The inflammation may be chemical or it may be infective, as a result of *Escherichia coli* in the gastrointestinal tract.

If the gallbladder becomes infected, it may fill with pus to form an empyema. Septicaemia may then ensue. Mucus secretion in the gallbladder may cause a mucocele, which is palpable as an enlarged gallbladder.

Necrosis and gangrene may result in perforation of the gallbladder, producing peritonitis.

If the gallbladder perforates into a part of the bowel, a cholecystoenteric fistula is created. Gallstones may then pass directly into the bowel and gallstone ileus may result.

3.31 Ascending cholangitis   Answers: B C D E

Ascending cholangitis is characterised by pain, pyrexia and jaundice. Obstruction of the bile ducts as a result of gallstones, bile duct stricture or carcinoma predisposes to infection, which ascends into the intrahepatic ducts. It may result in liver abscess. Invasive procedures, eg stent insertion, may introduce infection and cause cholangitis.

3.32 Carcinoma of the oesophagus   Answers: C D E

The classic presentation is dysphagia.

Investigations include a barium swallow, oesophagogastroduodenoscopy (OGD), which is very useful because biopsies can be taken if tumour is seen, and CT, which is used to determine the extent of spread and to assess operability. Spread is local, to surrounding tissue and local lymph nodes, and then further to the liver and lungs.

Radiotherapy is useful for squamous carcinoma.

Surgery is used for adenocarcinoma.

Chemotherapy is not used routinely.

3.33 Breast lump   Answers: D E

The skin changes in breast disease may be very subtle. Tethering of the skin or dimpling is suggestive of carcinoma. Fixation to the skin or deeper tissues also suggests carcinoma. Peau d'orange is pathognomonic of carcinoma.

When a lump is present, its characteristics (ie surface and texture) provide useful information. A fibroadenoma usually produces a discrete lump with a smooth surface. It is not fixed to the skin or deeper tissues. A lipoma is a soft mobile lump.

A cyst is smooth, discrete and very mobile.

Intraductal papilloma is not usually felt as a lump and tends to present as nipple discharge.

An abscess affects the skin and subcutaneous tissue. It is red, hot and tender. Collection of pus makes it fluctuant and it may point and then discharge. It is fixed to the skin, which may then become indurated.

Fat necrosis occurs after trauma to the breast. It forms a hard lump that may be fixed to the skin.

3.34 Splenic rupture   Answers: A C D E

A ruptured spleen presents with pain, tenderness and guarding in the left upper quadrant of the abdomen. Pain may be referred to the left shoulder. There is usually a history of trauma.

The following are the signs of internal haemorrhage:

- Hypotension/hypovolaemia
- Peritonitis, which may produce an ileus (if haemorrhage occurs into the peritoneal cavity)
- Abdominal distension
- Shifting dullness resulting from blood within the peritoneal cavity
- Fixed dullness, which may occur as a result of extraperitoneal blood loss.

Haematemesis does not occur because bleeding is not within the bowel.

The diagnosis may be confirmed by ultrasonography or CT.

Splenic rupture is treated by splenectomy with attention to immunisation and penicillin prophylaxis (see Question 4.34, Paper 4).

3.35 Renal calculi   Answers: B D E

Most renal calculi are idiopathic. The following factors predispose to their formation:

- Stagnation of urine: congenital or acquired obstruction
- Infection, eg urease-producing organisms such as *Proteus* species
- Dehydration/malnutrition
- Raised calcium levels, eg hyperparathyroidism, immobility
- Gout: uric acid
- Hyperoxaluria: calcium oxalate
- Cystinuria: cystine stones.

3.36 Renal trauma   Answers: C D E

Injury to the kidney commonly results in localised pain and haematuria, which may be macroscopic or microscopic. Hypotension may occur. The following are appropriate investigations:

- Intravenous urography
- Ultrasonography
- CT
- Arteriography.

Treatment is usually conservative. Close monitoring of urine output, pulse rate and blood pressure is required.

The patient should be followed up for several months after renal trauma because complications such as hypertension or renal failure may develop late. There may be persistent bleeding, which may necessitate nephrectomy.

3.37 Ulcerative colitis   Answers: A C E

Ulcerative colitis is an inflammatory bowel disease (along with Crohn's disease, amoebiasis, etc) affecting the colon. The cause is unknown but genetic and environmental factors have been implicated.

It is a mucosal disease that involves the rectum and spreads proximally. There is inflammation of the mucosa, crypt abscess formation and goblet cell depletion. Pseudopolyps occur where intact mucosa appears raised, adjacent to ulcerated mucosa.

In patients with pancolitis the risk of malignancy is significant and total colectomy is advised.

3.38 Complications of venous insufficiency   Answers: A B C E

Chronic venous insufficiency refers to the superficial venous system. It causes the following:

- Ankle flare resulting from venous hypertension
- Dilated calf 'blow-outs' caused by incompetent valves
- Superficial thrombophlebitis
- Eczema
- Pigmentation of the skin, usually over the medial aspect of the ankle; this may spread over the lower leg
- The skin may break down and ulcerate, especially over the medial malleolus; this may become infected and very painful; rarely, an ulcer undergoes malignant change, ie into a squamous cell carcinoma – this is called a Marjolin's ulcer
- Lipodermatosclerosis may occur; the skin becomes red, hot and tender
- Subcutaneous fibrosis causes stiffness of the ankle joint, which may cause fixed flexion.

Venous insufficiency is a complication of DVT.

3.39 Digital gangrene   Answers: A C E

Digital gangrene is caused by obstruction of blood flow to the tips of the fingers. It occurs in peripheral arterial disease. The causes include the following:

- Digital artery embolism, eg from the heart in atrial fibrillation or from a subclavian artery with atherosclerosis
- Thrombus formation
- Cervical rib: pressure on the sympathetic nerves may cause vasoconstriction; direct pressure on the subclavian artery would reduce blood flow
- Frostbite: where severe vasoconstriction causes hypoxia
- Blood disorders, eg cold agglutinins
- Vasculitis with vasospasm
- Raynaud's phenomenon
- Drugs, eg ergot derivatives or β blockers.

3.40 Anal fissure   Answers: A D E

Definition: An anal fissure is a longitudinal tear of the anal mucosa. It is exquisitely painful and patients often refuse anorectal examination. Defecation causes pain with prolonged burning and impairs healing. The most common site is the posterior anal margin. It occurs in infants, children and adults.

Externally, there may be a skin tag called a 'sentinel pile', where a previous fissure has healed.

The anal sphincter may increase in tone, causing constipation and bleeding, which is detected as a smear on the toilet paper. There may also be pruritus. Associated conditions are Crohn's disease, ulcerative colitis and TB.

3.41 Arterial embolus   Answers: A C D E

Definition: An embolus is the passage of a mass carried in the circulation. It produces its effects by lodging in smaller vessels and preventing oxygen and nutrients from reaching the tissues.

The following are the different types of embolus:

- Thrombus: this is the most common
- Fat: seen in fractures
- Air: occurs in neck or lung trauma or iatrogenically
- Nitrogen: caisson disease.

The following is the management of emboli:

- Anticoagulation to prevent extension and recurrence
- Thrombolysis: this is useful in patients in whom surgery is risky
- Surgical embolectomy.

The site of origin varies – commonly it arises in the heart and is caused by atrial fibrillation. It is the site where the embolus lodges rather than its site of origin that determines its effects. The size of the embolus will determine the site of impact and therefore its effects. The main effect of an embolus is ischaemia. The presence of a collateral circulation may therefore allow the tissue to remain viable.

An infected embolus, eg an embolus of vegetations from the heart, can lodge in an artery and cause a mycotic aneurysm.

3.42 Coronary artery bypass grafting   Answer: D

Coronary artery surgery may be performed on or off cardiopulmonary bypass. It is performed using the left internal mammary artery or a saphenous vein. Three- or four-vessel disease produces marked symptoms and hence surgery is very successful in relieving symptoms.

Investigations required before operation include the following:

- Chest radiograph
- Electrocardiogram (ECG)

- Exercise ECG
- Coronary angiography.

The operative mortality rate is 2–3%. In addition to the general complications, specific complications include strokes, neurological deficit and graft failure.

Surgery provides the following:

- Reduced morbidity with relief of symptoms in most cases
- Reduced mortality.

In patients with three- or four-vessel disease and severe symptoms, such as unstable angina, the mortality is reduced after surgery. However, in patients with one- or two-vessel disease, mortality is not improved by surgery.

3.43 Deep vein thrombosis prophylaxis   Answers: A B C

There is a significant risk of DVT postoperatively.

Predisposing factors include trauma, surgery, dehydration, immobilisation, malignancy, polycythaemia and the oral contraceptive pill. The risk is higher after major operations.

The following are the measures used to prevent DVT:

- Minimal trauma to the legs during handling of the patient
- Rehydration: increased blood viscosity predisposes to thrombosis
- Heparin (subcutaneous, 5000 IU twice daily)
- Elasticated compression stockings
- Pneumatic calf stockings during operations
- Early mobilisation
- Warfarin: but there is a risk of haemorrhage
- Intravenous dextran.

3.44 Surgical emphysema   Answers: B D

Surgical emphysema is caused by air tracking into subcutaneous tissues. Clinically there is swelling of the affected area with crepitus. It may be visible on a radiograph.

The causes are trauma and oesophageal rupture, and treatment is of the underlying cause. The surgical emphysema itself tends to resolve gradually with conservative treatment.

3.45 Anal pain   Answers: A C E

Lesions in the anal canal often present with pain, because anal skin is very sensitive.

Carcinoma can cause ulceration with bleeding and pain.

Perianal haematoma causes a localised inflammatory reaction that is painful.

Haemorrhoids are not painful as such, but it is their complications that cause pain. First-degree haemorrhoids are internal and not painful.

Anal warts cause irritation, itching and discomfort; they do not produce pain. An anal fissure is classically very painful, as fistula *in ano* can be, especially when infection occurs.

A perianal abscess causes pain and discomfort, especially on sitting.

3.46 Malignant melanoma   Answers: B D E

Most malignant melanomas arise in normal skin. Only a minority arise in a pre-existing mole. The prognosis depends on the depth of invasion. There are two classification systems used to determine prognosis:

1. Clark's level of invasion is based on the layer of skin penetrated: if the basement membrane is not penetrated the prognosis is good; invasion into the subcutaneous fat carries a very poor prognosis.
2. Breslow's classification uses the thickness of the tumour ('Breslow's index') to predict prognosis:

Depth of invasion (mm)	Risk
< 0.76	Low
0.76–1.5	Moderate
> 1.5	High

Most lesions are of the superficial spreading type. These have a better prognosis than the nodular type, which invade deeply.

Amelanotic lesions have a worse prognosis. This may be because they are diagnosed late or because they are inherently more aggressive.

Malignant melanomas spread via lymphatics to the regional lymph nodes, and via the bloodstream to the lungs, liver and brain.

3.47 Peripheral arterial disease

Answers: A B D E

Intermittent claudication is a sign of chronic lower limb ischaemia. As this worsens, it develops into rest pain and critical ischaemia. Critical ischaemia is arterial disease that threatens the viability of the foot or leg. It usually occurs gradually but can develop suddenly if there is thrombus or embolus occluding a vessel.

In acute critical ischaemia of the foot the classic features are the six 'Ps':

Pain
Pallor
Pulseless
Paraesthesia (numbness of the foot)
Paralysis (this is a late sign)
Perishing with cold.

Transient ischaemic attacks are a feature of ischaemic events in the brain that may result from carotid artery emboli.

Diabetes mellitus is associated with atherosclerosis. However, it is not a feature of peripheral arterial disease. Also, diabetic neuropathy results in injury and ulceration of the feet as a result of poor healing.

3.48 Tuberculosis

Answers: B C D E

The incidence of TB is increasing in the UK. It is caused by *Mycobacterium tuberculosis*, which can affect the lungs, bones, gastrointestinal tract, urinary tract and skin. It is characterised by granuloma formation and caseating necrosis. Pus forms slowly and results in the formation of an abscess. As the abscess forms slowly and there is no redness/inflammation, it is called a 'cold abscess'.

Infection of the spine can be devastating. It affects both the bone and the intervertebral disc spaces. Vertebral collapse may cause spinal cord compression, which requires surgical intervention.

TB spreads via the bloodstream to the genitourinary tract. Tuberculous epididymitis causes swelling of the scrotum, but symptoms may be mild and go unnoticed.

TB affecting the urinary tract causes frequency of micturition, as is seen in bacterial urinary tract infection.

3.49 Carcinoma of the tongue   Answers: C E

Carcinoma of the tongue occurs most commonly on the anterior two-thirds of the tongue. It is more common in men than in women. There is an association with pipe smoking, alcohol, leukoplakia, betel nut chewing and poor oral hygiene.

The presentation is of a nodule or ulcer. The tongue is covered in squamous epithelium and therefore the carcinoma is squamous in type. Spread occurs locally or by lymphatic drainage to the submental and cervical lymph nodes.

Prognosis depends on spread. If metastasis has occurred, the 5-year survival rate is only 18%.

Definitive treatment is by surgery, radiotherapy or both.

3.50 Prolapsed lumbar disc   Answers: B C D E

A prolapsed lumbar disc classically presents with back pain radiating to the buttock. There may be paraesthesia of the leg and muscle weakness.

At the affected level, reflexes are diminished, eg L3–4 – knee jerk; L5–S1 – ankle jerk. Cauda equina compression may cause urinary retention.

Treatment of a prolapsed disc is by the three 'Rs':

Rest
Removal
Rehabilitation

Improvement may occur after rest alone.

3.51 Bone metastases   Answers: A C E

This is a list well worth committing to memory. The sites of tumours commonly metastasising to bone include:

- breast
- thyroid
- bronchus
- prostate – remember that here they cause sclerotic lesions
- kidney.

Lesions are lytic (except prostate) and present as pathological fractures.

3.52 Intertrochanteric fracture of the femur   Answers: B C

Intertrochanteric fractures of the femur occur in elderly people, especially women who have osteoporosis, which weakens the bones. The fracture may be traumatic or pathological. The classic presentation is shortening of the leg and external rotation.

Intertrochanteric fractures are extracapsular, so they unite early with little risk of avascular necrosis. Treatment is by internal fixation to allow early mobilisation.

3.53 Antibiotics   Answers: A D E

Antibiotics are often used to prevent infection in surgery. A short sharp dosage is recommended (ie one to three doses given intravenously). Prolonged courses are not advantageous. The definitive treatment of an abscess is incision and drainage. Patients at high risk of infection during surgery require prophylactic antibiotics, eg patients with prosthetic heart valves, rheumatic heart disease, etc.

Cefuroxime (a second-generation cephalosporin) is active against entero-cocci and is often used for prophylaxis in cholecystectomy. In colorectal surgery, the major risk of infection is from bowel organisms, ie anaerobes; metronidazole is used for this. A cephalosporin is added for prophylaxis against aerobes.

3.54 Complications of urinary catheter insertion   Answers: C D E

The passage of a urinary catheter presents a risk of infection both on insertion and on removal. Epithelial damage allows access for bacteria to the circulation and septicaemia can result.

Artificial prostheses are particularly at risk. It is therefore very important to use aseptic technique.

Antibiotic cover (eg intramuscular gentamicin) can be used. Trauma during insertion may cause urethral bleeding.

Trauma to the prostate gland can cause acute prostatitis.

Renal calculi and chronic pyelonephritis are not a problem.

3.55 Preoperative investigations   Answers: A B E

The following are the urgent investigations required in large bowel obstruction:

- Full blood count
- Urea and electrolytes
- Creatinine
- Chest radiograph
- ECG.

These are the minimum requirements to facilitate safe anaesthesia.

Sigmoidoscopy is unlikely to alter the management.

A barium enema would cause delay. Laparotomy would still be required to relieve the obstruction. However, an instant barium enema may help to define the cause and level of obstruction. It is not advised in perforation.

3.56 Early postoperative complications   Answers: A C D E

In the first 12 hours after an operation, complications are those resulting from either anaesthesia or the surgery.

Complications of anaesthesia include the following:

- Drug reactions or side effects
- Trauma to the mouth or throat
- Postoperative nausea and vomiting
- Fluid imbalance: a fluid chart is essential to monitor fluid input and output. Bowel surgery causes loss of large amounts of fluid and hypovolaemia may result – this predisposes to acute renal failure. If excess fluid is given, cardiac failure may occur as a result of overloading
- Hypothermia: this can occur in bowel surgery where fluid loss is high and operations are long
- Lung atelectasis/aspiration: hypoxia may result and therefore attention must be paid to oxygenation.

Complications of surgery include the following:

- Reactionary haemorrhage: wound drainage is used to monitor any internal blood loss
- Hypothermia/sepsis
- Hypovolaemia: check urine output.

(See also Question 2.52, Paper 2.)

3.57 Total parenteral nutrition   Answers: B D

Total parenteral nutrition (TPN) is intravenous feeding; enteral nutrition is feeding via the gastrointestinal tract. TPN is indicated for malnourished patients in whom the gastrointestinal tract is not functioning, eg in obstruction.

Preoperatively, TPN is beneficial for patients who are severely malnourished, ie only about 5% of patients.

Postoperatively, TPN is beneficial in malnourished patients because it improves wound healing and is required to overcome the catabolic phase.

TPN solutions have high osmolalities and are therefore highly thrombophlebitic. They are therefore given via a central venous line into large veins where blood flow is high. The risks of central venous line insertion include haemorrhage, pneumothorax, air embolism and sepsis.

Enteral feeding is usually given via a fine-bore nasogastric tube. If this is not tolerated, a percutaneous endoscopic gastrostomy (PEG) can be used.

3.58 Rectal bleeding   Answers: A B D

Bleeding per rectum occurs in:

* diverticulitis
* carcinoma of the rectum or colon
* haemorrhoids
* Meckel's diverticulum
* intussusception
* colitis: blood and mucus are seen
* melaena: old dark blood from peptic ulceration.

Intussusception occurs when a segment of bowel 'telescopes' into the adjacent section. It is most common before the age of 2 years. Ileocaecal intussusception is the most common form. It presents with bowel obstruction and the blood passed per rectum is described as 'redcurrant jelly stool' and is pathognomonic. The management is an urgent barium enema which confirms the diagnosis and may even relieve the intussusception; if not, laparotomy is required.

Carcinoma of the oesophagus presents with faecal occult blood, but not blood on digital examination.

3.59 Bowel stricture   Answers: B C D

Bowel stricture is caused by a localised inflammatory response.
The causes include the following:

- Diverticular disease
- Neoplasia
- Crohn's disease
- Mesenteric ischaemia
- Slow-release potassium tablets

Gluten enteropathy, which causes loss of villi and Peutz–Jeghers syndrome, which is a cause of intestinal polyposis, do not cause bowel strictures.

3.60 Volvulus   Answers: A B C

Volvulus is a twisting of a loop of bowel. It usually occurs in elderly people and presents with abdominal distension and pain. Constipation may also be present. Complications are venous infarction or perforation, resulting in peritonitis. The sigmoid colon is most commonly affected, but the caecum can also be involved.

Investigations include a plain abdominal radiograph, which shows a dilated bowel – the sigmoid colon is commonly affected and has an inverted horseshoe appearance or a 'coffee-bean' appearance on the radiograph.

The following is the treatment:

- Insertion of a flatus tube to deflate the bowel
- Barium enema without preparation
- Surgery: laparotomy, sigmoid colectomy.

BEST OF FIVE AND MULTIPLE CHOICE QUESTIONS PAPER 4

60 questions: time allowed 2½ hours

Best of Five Questions
Mark your answers with a tick (True) in the box provided.

4.1   A 22-year-old woman has a firm, 1–2 cm mass in her left breast.
       There is no nipple discharge and no pain. No axillary
       lymphadenopathy is present. The overlying skin of the breast
       appears normal. Her urine pregnancy test is negative.
       Mammography confirms the presence of a rounded density,
       which has no microcalcifications, and reveals no lesions of the
       opposite breast. Which of the following is the most likely
       diagnosis?

❏   A   Cystosarcoma phyllodes
❏   B   Focus of fat necrosis
❏   C   Fibroadenoma
❏   D   Intraductal papilloma
❏   E   Infiltrating ductal carcinoma

4.2   An otherwise healthy 64-year-old woman with an unremarkable
       medical history has had increasing back pain and right hip pain
       for the last 3 years. The pain is worse at the end of the day. On
       physical examination she has bony enlargement of the distal
       interphalangeal joints. A radiograph of the spine reveals the
       presence of prominent osteophytes involving the vertebral
       bodies. There is sclerosis with narrowing of the joint space at the
       right acetabulum, seen on a radiograph of the pelvis. No
       biochemical abnormalities were detected on blood tests. Which
       of the following conditions is most likely to be affecting this
       patient?

❑ A Rheumatoid arthritis
❑ B Gout
❑ C Osteomyelitis
❑ D Osteoarthritis
❑ E Pseudogout

4.3 A 44-year-old man who is a heavy drinker experiences a bout of prolonged vomiting, followed by massive haematemesis. On physical examination in the A&E department, his vital signs are: pulse = 110 beats/min, blood pressure or BP = 80/40 mmHg, temperature = 36.8°C and respiratory rate = 22/min. Systemic examination is unremarkable. His stool is negative for occult blood. Which of the following conditions is responsible for the haematemesis?

❑ A Hiatal hernia
❑ B Mallory–Weiss syndrome
❑ C Oesophageal pulsion diverticulum
❑ D Barrett's oesophagus
❑ E Oesophageal stricture

4.4 A 30-year-old man has a right inguinal mass. On examination the left testis is palpated in the scrotum and is of normal size, but the right testis cannot be palpated in the scrotum. An ultrasound scan shows that the inguinal mass is consistent with a cryptorchid testis. Which of the following is the most appropriate treatment option to deal with this patient's testicular abnormality?

❑ A Put it into the scrotum surgically (orchiopexy)
❑ B Remove it
❑ C Remove it along with the opposite testis
❑ D Put the patient on testosterone
❑ E Perform a chromosome analysis

4.5 A 23-year-old healthy man undergoes physical examination before joining the army. On physical examination both his testes are palpable in the scrotum and the testes and scrotum are normal in size, with no masses palpable. However, the spermatic cord on the left has the feel of a 'bag of worms'. Laboratory studies show oligospermia. Which of the following conditions is this man most likely to have?

- ❏ A Testicular torsion
- ❏ B Hydrocele
- ❏ C Spermatocele
- ❏ D Seminoma
- ❏ E Varicocele

4.6   A 26-year-old man of African origin has acute onset of right upper quadrant abdominal pain. Abdominal ultrasonography reveals a dilated gallbladder with a thickened wall filled with calculi. A laparoscopic cholecystectomy is performed. Postoperatively, the gallbladder was opened to reveal the presence of several multifaceted 0.5–1 cm diameter dark, greenish-black gallstones. Which of the following underlying conditions is responsible for gallstone formation in this patient?

- ❏ A Hypercholesterolaemia
- ❏ B Sickle cell anaemia
- ❏ C Crohn's disease
- ❏ D Hyperparathyroidism
- ❏ E Primary biliary cirrhosis

4.7   A 55-year-old man with a history of chronic alcohol abuse presents in A&E with pain in the right and left upper quadrants. He has had bouts of abdominal pain in the past year. For the past month, he has had more frequent and worsening abdominal pain. Physical examination reveals right upper and left upper quandrant pain with guarding. An abdominal plain film radiograph reveals no free air, but there is extensive peritoneal fluid collection along with dilated loops of small bowel. An abdominal computed tomography (CT) scan reveals a 6–7 cm cystic mass in the tail of the pancreas. Which of the following is the most likely diagnosis?

- ❏ A Pancreatic pseudocyst
- ❏ B Islet cell adenoma
- ❏ C Acute pancreatitis
- ❏ D Metastatic carcinoma
- ❏ E Pancreatic adenocarcinoma

4.8 An 80-year-old woman falls on her outstretched hand and is brought to A&E with a painful and deformed wrist that looks like a dinner fork. A radiograph shows a dorsally displaced, dorsally angulated fracture of the distal radius. There is also an associated fracture of the ulnar styloid process. Neurological examination is unremarkable. Which of the following is the most appropriate treatment for this fracture?

- ❑ A Open reduction and internal fixation
- ❑ B Intramedullary rod
- ❑ C Skeletal traction
- ❑ D Closed reduction and short arm cast
- ❑ E Closed reduction and long arm cast

4.9 A 4–week-old, previously healthy baby boy begins to exhibit forceful vomiting after each meal. Before this he had been gaining weight normally. Which of the following disorders is the most likely cause for his vomiting?

- ❑ A Congenital duodenal atresia
- ❑ B Hirschsprung's disease
- ❑ C Tracheo-oesophageal fistula
- ❑ D Pyloric stenosis
- ❑ E Necrotising enterocolitis

4.10 A 48-year-old woman, on a return visit to the surgical outpatient clinic after a right-sided mastectomy for carcinoma of breast, complains that she cannot reach as far forward (such as to reach for a door knob) as she could before the operation. Physical examination reveals that the vertebral (medial) border of the patient's scapula projects posteriorly and is closer to the midline on the side of surgery. The nerve injury that caused these symptoms is to:

- ❑ A The axillary
- ❑ B The long thoracic
- ❑ C The musculocutaneous
- ❑ D The radial
- ❑ E The suprascapular

4.11 A 65-year-old female patient says that she has pain in her groin and upper thigh. Upon examination, a lump is palpable below the inguinal ligament lateral to its attachment to the pubic tubercle. You suspect that this may be a hernia passing through:

- ☐ A The adductor hiatus
- ☐ B The femoral canal
- ☐ C The obturator canal
- ☐ D The deep inguinal ring
- ☐ E The superficial inguinal ring

4.12 An 80-year-old woman fell from stairs and fractured the neck of her right femur. Fracture of the femoral neck may lead to avascular necrosis of the femoral head as a result of the interruption of which artery?

- ☐ A First perforating branch of the deep femoral
- ☐ B Inferior epigastric
- ☐ C Internal pudendal
- ☐ D Medial circumflex femoral
- ☐ E Lateral circumflex femoral

4.13 A 24-year-old female trainee solicitor has had difficulty concentrating on her job for the past 2 months. She complains that the work area is too hot. She seems nervous and has a fine tremor. She has been eating more but has lost 4 kg in the past month. On physical examination her temperature is 37.8°C, pulse 110 beats/min, respiratory rate 18/min and BP 145/85 mmHg. She has a wide staring gaze and lid lag. Which of the following laboratory findings is most likely to be present in this woman?

- ☐ A Decreased plasma insulin
- ☐ B Decreased iodine uptake
- ☐ C Increased free thyroxine
- ☐ D Increased ACTH (adrenocorticotrophic hormone)
- ☐ E Increased calcitonin

4.14   A 65-year-old man with a past history of hypertension, hypercholesterolaemia, peripheral vascular disease and bilateral carotid endarterectomy developed sudden pain in his right foot with a dusky colour change. On examination in A&E he had a cold, blue, painful foot with absent dorsalis pedis and posterior tibial pulse. Which of the following will be the most appropriate investigation for this patient?

- ❑   A   CT of the head and neck
- ❑   B   CT of the abdomen
- ❑   C   Echocardiogram
- ❑   D   Lateral radiograph of the cervical spine
- ❑   E   Lower limb angiography

4.15   A 68-year-old woman arrives in A&E with a 2-day history of severe right upper quadrant abdominal pain. On arrival she is confused and hypotensive. Her vital signs are pulse 115 beats/min, BP 95/40 mmHg, respiratory rate 22/min and temperature 40°C. There was severe tenderness along with muscle guarding in the right upper quadrant. Past history was positive for gallstones. Laboratory investigations showed a white cell count (WCC) of 25 000/mm³, bilirubin 6 mg/dL and alkaline phosphatase 1000 U/L. Abdominal ultrasonography showed multiple stones in the thick-walled gallbladder, with dilated intrahepatic ducts and a dilated common bile duct with a diameter of 2.4 cm. The patient was started on intravenous fluids and antibiotics. What will be the next most appropriate step in her management?

- ❑   A   Elective cholecystectomy
- ❑   B   Emergency cholecystectomy
- ❑   C   Emergency decompression of the common bile duct with ERCP (endoscopic retrograde cholangiopancreatography)
- ❑   D   Emergency surgical exploration of the common bile duct
- ❑   E   Masterly inactivity

Multiple Choice Questions
Mark your answers with a tick (True) or a cross (False) in the box provided. Leave the box blank for 'Don't know'. Do not look at the answers until you have completed the whole question paper.

4.16   Carcinoma of the breast:

❏ A   Is associated with Paget's disease of the nipple
❏ B   May be hormone dependent
❏ C   Should be treated by mastectomy
❏ D   May be asymptomatic
❏ E   Is detected by mammography on the NHS breast-screening programme

4.17   The carcinoid syndrome:

❏ A   May include valvular lesions of the heart
❏ B   May be treated with antibiotics
❏ C   Is characterised by flushing and diarrhoea
❏ D   Can occur only with liver metastases
❏ E   May present as appendicitis

4.18   Osteoarthritis of the hip can be treated with:

❏ A   Total knee replacement
❏ B   Steroids
❏ C   Arthrodesis
❏ D   Osteotomy
❏ E   Hemiarthroplasty

4.19   Dukes' staging of colorectal carcinoma:

❏ A   Involves assessment of lymph node spread
❏ B   Requires assessment of the depth of tumour penetration through the wall of the bowel
❏ C   Involves assessment of the presence or absence of metastases in distant organs
❏ D   Is made *post mortem*
❏ E   Requires measurement of the distances between the tumour and the resection lines

4.20 Femoral hernia:

- A Frequently becomes strangulated
- B Is more common in men than in women
- C Causes swelling of the lower limb
- D May be confused with an enlarged lymph node
- E Is more common than inguinal hernia

4.21 Gallstones:

- A Are usually formed in the bile ducts
- B Have been found in the stools
- C Are causally related to carcinoma of the gallbladder
- D Are usually radio-opaque
- E Can cause acute pancreatitis

4.22 In ureteric obstruction caused by a calculus, an intravenous urogram would be expected to show:

- A Normal excretion in the non-affected kidney
- B Delayed excretion in the affected kidney
- C Enlargement of the affected kidney
- D Contraction of the unaffected kidney
- E The site of obstruction

4.23 A full-thickness burn of the right leg:

- A Is estimated to represent 5% of the entire body surface area
- B May cause a peptic ulcer
- C May result in thrombosis
- D Is treated by resuscitation with intravenous fluids
- E Should be covered with ice

4.24 Causes of hypotension in adults include:

- A An upper gastrointestinal bleed
- B Intracranial bleeding
- C Myocardial infarction
- D Infarction of the small bowel
- E Systemic infection with Gram-negative organisms

4.25   Subphrenic abscesses:

- ❏ A   Are best treated by antibiotics
- ❏ B   Occur after a perforated peptic ulcer
- ❏ C   May be associated with a pleural effusion on the same side
- ❏ D   Cause hiccoughs
- ❏ E   Should not be treated by aspiration alone

4.26   Clinical features typical of acute appendicitis include:

- ❏ A   Fetor oris
- ❏ B   Fever
- ❏ C   Pain in the right shoulder
- ❏ D   Guarding in the left iliac fossa
- ❏ E   Anorexia

4.27   In Bell's palsy:

- ❏ A   Patients may complain of impairment of taste
- ❏ B   There is unilateral facial weakness
- ❏ C   There is unilateral loss of sensation of the skin
- ❏ D   Herpes zoster is the cause
- ❏ E   The voice is hoarse

4.28   Avascular necrosis occurs in:

- ❏ A   Fracture through the waist of the scaphoid
- ❏ B   Dislocation of the lunate bone
- ❏ C   Subcapital fracture of the femoral neck
- ❏ D   Steroid therapy
- ❏ E   Caisson disease

4.29   Gynaecomastia occurs in:

- ❏ A   Carcinoma of the prostate
- ❏ B   Chronic liver disease
- ❏ C   Carcinoma of the breast
- ❏ D   Peptic ulcer disease
- ❏ E   Bronchial carcinoma

4.30   Which of the following conditions may predispose to the development of paralytic ileus?

❑   A   Laparotomy
❑   B   Potassium deficiency
❑   C   Lumbar sympathectomy
❑   D   Fracture of lumbar vertebrae
❑   E   Calcium deficiency

4.31   In the trauma situation, after a road traffic accident (RTA):

❑   A   Screening radiographs should include cervical spine, chest and pelvis
❑   B   The treatment of a tension pneumothorax is immediate thoracotomy
❑   C   Bleeding from a wound in the thigh should be treated by direct pressure on the wound
❑   D   Open pneumothorax is treated with an occlusive dressing over the wound
❑   E   Pulse oximetry measures oxygen pressure

4.32   The causes of an acutely painful swelling in the scrotum of an 11-year-old boy include:

❑   A   Epididymo-orchitis
❑   B   Torsion of the testes
❑   C   Hydrocele
❑   D   Seminoma
❑   E   Varicocele

4.33   Intussusception:

❑   A   In infants usually requires resection of the bowel
❑   B   Presents with bowel obstruction
❑   C   Causes bleeding from the bowel
❑   D   Is twisting of the bowel
❑   E   Can be treated with a barium enema

4.34   Splenectomy:

- ❏ A   Is indicated in congenital spherocytosis
- ❏ B   Is of value in splenomegaly caused by myelofibrosis
- ❏ C   Should be preceded by *Haemophilus influenzae* immunisation
- ❏ D   May be complicated by gastric dilatation
- ❏ E   Is followed by administration of long-term penicillin

4.35   The following occur with gastro-oesophageal reflux:

- ❏ A   Pneumonia
- ❏ B   Oesophageal stricture
- ❏ C   Iron deficiency anaemia
- ❏ D   Polyneuritis
- ❏ E   Pernicious anaemia

4.36   Investigation of Crohn's disease often reveals:

- ❏ A   A lead-pipe colon on barium enema
- ❏ B   Increased uptake on a white cell scan
- ❏ C   Rose-thorn ulcers
- ❏ D   Strictures
- ❏ E   Toxic megacolon

4.37   Common signs of obstructive jaundice include:

- ❏ A   Dark stools
- ❏ B   Dark urine
- ❏ C   Splenomegaly
- ❏ D   Itching
- ❏ E   A palpable gallbladder

4.38   A hydrocele:

- ❏ A   May be pre-malignant
- ❏ B   May occur after repair of a hernia
- ❏ C   Occurs in the processus vaginalis
- ❏ D   Causes infertility
- ❏ E   Is reducible

4.39 Recurrent anal fistulae are associated with:

- ☐ A Crohn's disease
- ☐ B Ulcerative colitis
- ☐ C Carcinoma
- ☐ D Peutz–Jeghers syndrome
- ☐ E Diverticular disease

4.40 A patient aged 65 years presents with severe abdominal pain radiating to the back, abdominal distension and hypotension. The probable diagnosis is:

- ☐ A A leaking aortic aneurysm
- ☐ B Renal colic
- ☐ C Acute appendicitis
- ☐ D Acute pancreatitis
- ☐ E Pelvic inflammatory disease

4.41 Buerger's disease or thrombophlebitis obliterans:

- ☐ A Affects young men
- ☐ B Is confined to smokers
- ☐ C Involves upper limb and lower limb arteries
- ☐ D Is usually associated with Raynaud's phenomenon
- ☐ E Affects the veins as well as the arteries

4.42 In anal fissures the treatment is:

- ☐ A Laxatives
- ☐ B Anal dilatation
- ☐ C Examination under anaesthetic
- ☐ D Often not required
- ☐ E Excision of the fissure

4.43 Carpal tunnel syndrome may result in:

- ☐ A Hypothenar wasting
- ☐ B Wasting of the interossei
- ☐ C Reduced sensation over the index finger
- ☐ D Positive Tinel's sign
- ☐ E Pain in the forearm

4.44   A peptic ulcer:

☐   A   Occurs only in the stomach
☐   B   May give rise to haemorrhage
☐   C   May cause obstruction in the duodenum
☐   D   Is always associated with stress
☐   E   May be associated with hyperparathyroidism

4.45   Meckel's diverticulum:

☐   A   Is seen in 20% of the population
☐   B   Is a remnant of the vitello-intestinal duct
☐   C   Is a small appendix
☐   D   Is associated with peptic ulceration
☐   E   May present as acute appendicitis

4.46   Acute extradural haemorrhage:

☐   A   Causes a rise in pulse rate and a fall in BP
☐   B   Causes a fall in pulse rate and a rise in BP
☐   C   Results in hemiparesis
☐   D   Is associated with a dilated pupil on the side of the injury
☐   E   Can be distinguished from subdural haemorrhage by CT

4.47   Carcinoma of the caecum:

☐   A   Presents early with bloody diarrhoea
☐   B   Is treated by right hemicolectomy
☐   C   Is associated with microcytic anaemia
☐   D   Is associated with Crohn's disease
☐   E   Is diagnosed with sigmoidoscopy

4.48   Which of the following symptoms and signs are suggestive of paralytic ileus?

☐   A   Abdominal distension
☐   B   Hyperactive bowel sounds
☐   C   Vomiting
☐   D   Colicky abdominal pain
☐   E   Gas and fluid levels in dilated loops of small bowel on a radiograph

4.49   Dysphagia:

☐ A   Means difficulty in swallowing
☐ B   Means difficulty in speaking
☐ C   May occur in a patient who has had a stroke
☐ D   Is associated with carcinoma of the oesophagus
☐ E   Occurs in pyloric stenosis

4.50   Diverticular disease of the colon:

☐ A   May present with pneumaturia
☐ B   Always occurs in the jejunum
☐ C   Is common in western societies
☐ D   May present with massive bleeding
☐ E   Is a causative factor in the development of carcinoma of the colon

4.51   Hepatitis B:

☐ A   Is transmitted by the faecal–oral route
☐ B   Vaccine should be given to 'at-risk' healthcare workers
☐ C   Predisposes to hepatocellular carcinoma
☐ D   May cause liver cirrhosis
☐ E   Is an RNA virus

4.52   A direct inguinal hernia:

☐ A   Is usually congenital
☐ B   May contain bowel, omentum or bladder
☐ C   May occur with an indirect hernia
☐ D   Protrudes through the posterior wall of the inguinal canal, lateral
        to the inferior epigastric vessels
☐ E   Has a high risk of strangulation

4.53   In pancreatitis:

☐ A   Antibiotics are mandatory
☐ B   The clinical picture is a reliable indicator of prognosis
☐ C   Treatment is conservative
☐ D   Laparotomy may be indicated
☐ E   A rise in serum amylase is diagnostic

4.54   A carbuncle:

- ❑ A   Is associated with glycosuria
- ❑ B   Is commonly found on the palm of the hand
- ❑ C   Is commonly found on the neck
- ❑ D   Forms an area of necrosis with multiple sinuses
- ❑ E   Is best treated with systemic antibiotics

4.55   Heparin:

- ❑ A   Is given intravenously in the prophylaxis of deep vein thrombosis (DVT)
- ❑ B   May cause osteomalacia
- ❑ C   Is reversible with protamine
- ❑ D   Has a half-life of 12 hours
- ❑ E   Action is monitored by the international normalised ratio (INR)

4.56   Hyperhidrosis:

- ❑ A   Is dryness of the skin
- ❑ B   Is associated with an increase in the number of eccrine glands
- ❑ C   Does not occur in the palms
- ❑ D   Can be eliminated by a sympathectomy
- ❑ E   Classically affects young women

4.57   Pseudomembranous colitis:

- ❑ A   Is caused by *Clostridium perfringens*
- ❑ B   May occur after only one dose of an antibiotic
- ❑ C   May occur weeks after antibiotic treatment
- ❑ D   May occur after treatment with cephalosporins
- ❑ E   Is treated with intravenous metronidazole

4.58   Thyroid carcinoma:

- ❑ A   Of the papillary type usually affects young adults
- ❑ B   Presents as a lump in the neck that moves on swallowing
- ❑ C   Of the anaplastic type carries the best prognosis
- ❑ D   Of the medullary type is a tumour of parafollicular cells
- ❑ E   Typically causes thyroid dysfunction

4.59 **With regard to kidney transplantation:**

- ❏ A It is offered only to patients aged under 50 years
- ❏ B The transplant is placed extraperitoneally
- ❏ C Urine output is monitored to detect rejection
- ❏ D Immunosuppression is required
- ❏ E A urinary tract infection is a contraindication

4.60 **The level of amylase in serum is typically raised in patients with:**

- ❏ A Acute pancreatitis
- ❏ B Acute appendicitis
- ❏ C Renal failure
- ❏ D Perforated peptic ulcer
- ❏ E Acute cholecystitis

———————————————— **END** ————————————————

**Go over your answers until your time is up. Correct answers
and teaching notes are overleaf.**

BEST OF FIVE AND MULTIPLE CHOICE QUESTIONS PAPER 4
Answers

The correct answer options for each question are given below.

4.1	C		4.31	A C D
4.2	D		4.32	A B
4.3	B		4.33	B C E
4.4	B		4.34	A B C D E
4.5	E		4.35	A B C
4.6	B		4.36	B C D
4.7	A		4.37	B D E
4.8	E		4.38	B C
4.9	D		4.39	A B C
4.10	B		4.40	A D
4.11	B		4.41	A B C E
4.12	D		4.42	A B D
4.13	C		4.43	C D E
4.14	E		4.44	B C E
4.15	C		4.45	B D E
4.16	A B D E		4.46	B C D E
4.17	A C E		4.47	B C
4.18	C D		4.48	A C E
4.19	A B		4.49	A C D
4.20	A D		4.50	A C D
4.21	B C E		4.51	B C D
4.22	A B C E		4.52	B C
4.23	B C D		4.53	C D
4.24	A C D E		4.54	A C D E
4.25	B C D		4.55	C
4.26	A B E		4.56	D E
4.27	A B		4.57	B C D
4.28	A B C D E		4.58	A B D
4.29	B E		4.59	B C D E
4.30	A B D		4.60	A C D E

BEST OF FIVE AND MULTIPLE CHOICE QUESTIONS PAPER 4
Answers and Teaching Notes

4.1 C: Fibroadenoma

Fibroadenoma is the most common benign tumour of the female breast. Occurring at any age within the reproductive period of life, fibroadenomas are somewhat more common before age 30. They are frequently multiple and bilateral. The epithelium of the fibroadenoma is hormonally responsive, and a slight increase in size may occur during the late phase of each menstrual cycle. An increase in size caused by lactational changes or, not uncommonly, infarction and inflammation may lead to a fibroadenoma mimicking carcinoma during pregnancy. Regression usually occurs after menopause.

Cystosarcoma phyllodes, similar to fibroadenomas, arise from intralobular stroma. Although they can occur at any age, most present in the sixth decade, 10–20 years later than the average presentation of a fibroadenoma. Most present as palpable masses, but a few are detected mammographically. Cystosarcoma phyllodes must be excised with wide margins or by mastectomy to avoid the high risk of local recurrences. Axillary lymph node dissection is not indicated because the incidence of nodal metastases, as for other stromal malignancies, is exceedingly small.

Fat necrosis can present as a painless palpable mass, skin thickening or retraction, a mammographic density or mammographic calcifications. The majority of women will give a history of trauma or prior surgery.

Large duct papillomas are usually solitary and situated in the lactiferous sinuses of the nipple. Small duct papillomas are commonly multiple and located deeper within the ductal system.

A carcinoma would not be expected to be discrete, and age 25 is quite young for carcinoma.

4.2   D: Osteoarthritis

Degenerative osteoarthritis is a common and progressive condition that becomes more frequent and symptomatic with ageing (primary osteoarthritis). There is erosion and loss of articular cartilage. The term 'osteoarthritis' implies an inflammatory disease. However, although inflammatory cells may be present, osteoarthritis is considered to be an intrinsic disease of articular cartilage in which biochemical and metabolic alterations result in its breakdown. Osteoarthritis is an insidious disease. Patients with primary disease are usually asymptomatic until they are in their 50s. If a young patient has significant manifestations of osteoarthritis (secondary osteoarthritis), a search for some underlying cause should be made. Characteristic symptoms include deep, achy pain that worsens with use, morning stiffness, crepitus and limitation of range of movement.

Impingement on spinal foramina by osteophytes results in cervical and lumbar nerve root compression with radicular pain, muscle spasms, muscle atrophy and neurological deficits. Typically, only one or a few joints are involved, except in the uncommon generalised variant. The joints commonly involved include the hips, knees, lower lumbar and cervical vertebrae, proximal and distal interphalangeal joints of the fingers, first carpometacarpal joints and first tarsometatarsal joints of the feet. Characteristic in women, but not in men, are Heberden nodes in the fingers, representing prominent osteophytes at the distal interphalangeal joints.

Rheumatoid arthritis typically involves the small joints of the hands and feet most severely, and there is a destructive pannus that leads to marked joint deformity. A gouty arthritis is more likely to be accompanied by swelling and deformity, with joint destruction. The pain is not related to usage.

Osteomyelitis represents an ongoing infection that produces marked bone deformity, not just joint narrowing. Pseudogout, or calcium pyrophosphate dihydrate deposition disease, is more often a disease of elderly people, accompanied by meniscal calcification and joint space narrowing. There can be acute attacks with marked pain. The knees are most often involved.

4.3   B: Mallory–Weiss syndrome

Longitudinal tears in the oesophagus at the oesophagogastric junction or gastric cardia are termed 'Mallory–Weiss tears' and are thought to be the consequence of severe retching or vomiting. They are encountered most commonly in people with alcohol problems, in whom they are attributed to episodes of excessive vomiting in the setting of an alcoholic stupor. Normally, a reflex relaxation of the musculature of the gastrointestinal tract precedes the anti-peristaltic wave of contraction. During episodes of prolonged vomiting, it is speculated that this reflex relaxation fails to occur. The refluxing gastric contents suddenly overwhelm the contraction of the musculature at the gastric inlet, and massive dilatation with tearing of the stretched wall ensues.

Hiatus hernia is characterised by separation of the diaphragmatic crura and widening of the space between the muscular crura and the oesophageal wall. Two anatomical patterns are recognised: the axial, or sliding hernia, and the non-axial, or para-oesophageal hiatus hernia.

The sliding hernia constitutes 95% of cases; protrusion of the stomach above the diaphragm creates a bell-shaped dilatation, bounded below by the diaphragmatic narrowing. In para-oesophageal hernias, a separate portion of the stomach, usually along the greater curvature, enters the thorax through the widened foramen. Bleeding with hiatus hernia is not usually massive. Diverticula of the oesophagus do not often bleed. Barrett mucosa is associated with reflux with inflammation and possible ulceration, but bleeding is not usually massive.

Strictures of the oesophagus result from scarring, typically with reflux or with scleroderma. It is a chronic process without massive haemorrhage.

4.4   B: Remove it

At the age of 30 the cryptorchid testis no longer functions and presents a risk for subsequent development of seminoma. The earlier in life that an orchiopexy is performed, generally under the age of 5, the more likely that the testis will function properly.

The testis has been out of place too long to retain any function of spermato-genesis. It is now atrophic with few remaining germ cells and minimal, if any, spermatogenesis. Therefore, orchiopexy is not a good option. The opposite testis will not be affected by the cryptorchid testis and hence must not be removed. The patient still has one good testis. Even with bilateral cryptorchidism, the Leydig cells of the testicular interstitium continue to function and produce testosterone, so this patient does not need testos-terone. Chromosome analysis is indicated if the patient had a chromosomal defect. If this were testicular feminisation with androgen insensitivity, the phenotype would be female. If he had Klinefelter syndrome, the testes would be small and in the scrotum.

4.5   E: Varicocele

Varicoceles are dilated veins in the scrotum. The condition affects 10–15% of all men and the typical patient is aged between 15 and 35 years; it is very rare in old people. This condition occurs on the left side in 85% of patients, on both sides in about 11% and on the right side in only about 4%. The dilated veins cause a rise in temperature of a few degrees in the testicle, which for a long period may cause oligospermia, leading to infertility.

Torsion is an acute emergency because the arterial blood supply to the testis is cut off. A hydrocele may produce an enlargement that has smooth borders. Hydroceles generally do not affect the sperm count. A spermatocele is usually a small, circumscribed mass and does not affect the sperm count. A seminoma usually produces a firm mass lesion.

4.6   B: Sickle cell anaemia

There are two main types of gallstones. In the west, about 80% are cholesterol stones, containing more than 50% crystalline cholesterol monohydrate. The remainder are composed predominantly of bilirubin calcium salts and are designated as pigment stones. The patient in this question is of African origin, which points to sickle cell disease, which when it results in haemolysis leads to hyperbilirubinaemia; this predisposes to pigment stone formation. The stones in this question are typical pigment stones.

Pure cholesterol stones are pale yellow and round to ovoid, and have a finely granular, hard external surface; on transection this reveals a glistening radiating crystalline palisade. Such stones are usually seen in hypercholesterolaemia. Yellow-to-green stones, mainly cholesterol stones, are more likely to form when there is a reduction in bile acids from decreased enterohepatic circulation with Crohn's disease. Hypercalcaemia leads to gallstone formation, with increased calcium combined with cholesterol to produce yellow–white stones. Primary biliary cirrhosis produces an increase in serum cholesterol with cholelithiasis in about 15% of cases, mainly cholesterol stones that are yellow to green.

4.7   A: Pancreatic pseudocyst

Pseudocysts are localised collections of necrotic–haemorrhagic material rich in pancreatic enzymes. Such cysts lack an epithelial lining (hence the prefix 'pseudo'), and they account for about 75% of cysts in the pancreas. Pseudocysts usually arise after an episode of acute pancreatitis, often in the setting of chronic alcoholic pancreatitis. Traumatic injury to the abdomen can also give rise to them.

Islet cell adenomas are not cystic, and are often so small that they are difficult to image. Most are non-functional, but some may secrete hormones such as insulin and gastrin. Acute pancreatitis is a group of reversible lesions characterised by inflammation of the pancreas, ranging in severity from oedema and fat necrosis to parenchymal necrosis with severe haemorrhage. Full-blown acute pancreatitis is a medical emergency of the first magnitude. These patients usually have the sudden calamitous onset of an 'acute abdomen' which must be differentiated from diseases such as ruptured acute appendicitis, perforated peptic ulcer, acute cholecystitis with rupture and occlusion of mesenteric vessels with infarction of the bowel.

Characteristically, the pain is constant and intense, and is often referred to the upper back. Metastases are most often multiple solid masses. A primary adenocarcinoma of the pancreas is usually a solid mass. Development of pancreatic adenocarcinoma is not related to alcoholism. About 60% of cancers of the pancreas arise in the head of the gland, 15% in the body and 5% in the tail; in 20%, the neoplasm diffusely involves the entire gland. Carcinomas of the pancreas are usually hard, stellate, grey–white, poorly defined masses

4.8   E: Closed reduction and long arm cast

This patient has a Colles' fracture, which typically can be reduced well with closed manipulation. Casting should immobilise both the wrist and the elbow, so a long arm cast is needed.

Open reduction and internal fixation will provide a very nice result, but it will be an unnecessarily expensive and invasive way of dealing with this fracture. An intramedullary rod is usually used for fractures of the shafts of long bones. Skeletal traction could reduce the deformity but it will affect the future function of the hand.

4.9   D: Pyloric stenosis

Male sex, time after birth and symptoms are all quite typical. Pyloric stenosis is a condition that exhibits the genetic feature called the 'threshold of liability', in which boys are more likely to have the disease (lower threshold) if born into a family with affected girls (higher threshold and, thus, more genetic tendencies for the disease to pass on).

Congenital duodenal atresia would have caused problems much earlier in life. Half of all occurrences of duodenal atresia are seen in association with Down syndrome (trisomy 21). Hirschsprung's disease is colonic dilatation resulting from an aganglionic segment. There are several variations of tracheo-oesophageal fistula, which can include oesophageal atresia. The vomiting should be apparent from birth, not a month later. Tracheo-oesophageal fistula is often present with other congenital anomalies. An example is the VATER association. A child with necrotising enterocolitis is usually very sick.

4.10 B: Long thoracic

Injury to the long thoracic nerve denervates serratus anterior, meaning that there will be no muscle protracting the scapula and counteracting trapezius and the rhomboids, powerful retractors of the scapula. The long thoracic nerve is derived from the nerve roots of C5–7; this nerve is particularly vulnerable to iatrogenic injury during surgical procedures because it is located on the superficial side of serratus anterior.

The axillary nerve innervates teres minor and deltoid. It wraps around the surgical neck of the humerus and is endangered by fractures of the surgical neck. If the axillary nerve were damaged and deltoid were denervated, the patient would be unable to abduct her or his upper limb beyond 15–20°.

The musculocutaneous nerve innervates biceps brachi, coracobrachialis and brachialis. If this nerve were disrupted, the patient would be unable to flex her or his forearm, and have weakened arm flexion.

The radial nerve innervates extensors of the forearm and triceps brachi – if this nerve were injured, the patient would no longer be able to extend his or her forearm, but only have a slightly weakened arm extension (latissimus is the powerful extensor of the arm). Finally, the suprascapular nerve innervates supraspinatus – the muscle that initiates abduction. Damage to this nerve would prevent the patient from starting to abduct his or her arm.

4.11 B: Femoral canal

The patient has a femoral hernia. Central to understanding the anatomy of a femoral hernia is understanding of the relationships in the femoral triangle. The femoral triangle is an area bounded superiorly by the inguinal ligament, laterally by sartorius and medially by the medial edge of adductor longus. There are two main things in the femoral triangle: the femoral nerve and the femoral sheath, which encloses the femoral artery, vein and canal. The femoral nerve is at the lateral edge of the triangle – it is not enclosed by the femoral sheath. Medial to the femoral nerve, you can see the femoral sheath, enclosing the artery, vein and canal, in that order from lateral to medial. The femoral canal is the most medial structure in the triangle. It opens up to the abdominal cavity through the femoral ring, so the abdominal contents might herniate through that ring and into the femoral canal. As the hernia is inferior to the inguinal ligament, it has entered the femoral canal.

The other common hernia sites listed among the answers are the superficial and deep inguinal rings. However, these hernias would be palpated near the superficial inguinal ring, which is superolateral to the pubic tubercle. The adductor hiatus is a space in the adductor magnus that allows the femoral vessels to pass through and reach the posterior surface of the leg, where they become the popliteal vessels. Finally, the obturator canal is the space in the obturator foramen through which the obturator nerve and vessels travel.

4.12 D: Medial circumflex femoral

It is important to remember that the medial circumflex femoral artery supplies blood to the femoral neck. During fractures of the femoral neck, this artery may be ruptured, and the femoral neck will be deprived of blood. The perforating branches of the deep femoral artery supply the posterior compartment of the thigh, including the hamstrings. The inferior epigastric artery is a branch of the external iliac artery that supplies the lower abdominal wall. The internal pudendal artery is the major source of blood to the perineum. The lateral circumflex femoral artery supplies the lateral thigh and hip. Although it contributes to the circulation around the hip, the primary supply to the head of the femur usually comes from the medial femoral circumflex.

4.13 C: Increased free thyroxine

The patient has features suggestive of hyperthyroidism. Therefore, there will be increased free thyroxine (T_4). The clinical manifestations of hyperthyroidism are protean and include changes referable to the hypermetabolic state induced by excess thyroid hormone, as well as those related to overactivity of the sympathetic nervous system (ie an increase in the β-adrenergic 'tone'). Excessive levels of thyroid hormone result in an increase in the basal metabolic rate.

The skin of thyrotoxic patients tends to be soft, warm and flushed because of increased blood flow and peripheral vasodilatation to increase heat loss. Heat intolerance is common. Sweating is increased because of higher levels of calorigenesis. An increased basal metabolic rate also results in characteristic weight loss despite increased appetite. Tachycardia, palpitations and cardiomegaly are common.

Arrhythmias, particularly atrial fibrillation, occur frequently and are more common in older patients. In the neuromuscular system, overactivity of the sympathetic nervous system produces tremor, hyperactivity, emotional lability, anxiety, inability to concentrate and insomnia. Proximal muscle weakness is common with decreased muscle mass (thyroid myopathy).

Ocular changes often call attention to hyperthyroidism. A wide, staring gaze and lid lag are present because of sympathetic overstimulation of the levator palpebrae superioris. However, true thyroid ophthalmopathy associated with proptosis is a feature seen only in Graves' disease. In the gastrointestinal system, sympathetic hyperstimulation of the gut results in hypermotility, malabsorption and diarrhoea. The iodine uptake is increased, and not decreased, with the hyperfunctioning thyroid.

Decreased plasma insulin would indicate diabetes mellitus. This patient's symptoms are not related to Cushing syndrome or Cushing's disease, so ACTH levels should be normal. Calcitonin may be increased with medullary thyroid cancers, but is not a feature of hyperthyroidism.

4.14 E: Lower limb angiography

Lower limb angiography will indicate the site of occlusion of the arterial supply in this patient. This will help to formulate a treatment strategy such as vascular exploration and embolectomy or fasciotomy.

As there is no history of trauma to the abdomen or head and neck CT is not indicated. The same holds true for a cervical spine radiograph. An echocardiogram can be done in this patient to exclude the possibility of a cardiac source of embolisation; however, priority will be lower limb angiography so that the foot can be salvaged.

4.15 C: Emergency decompression of the common bile duct with ERCP

This patient has the classic presentation of acute ascending cholangitis. The condition is usually seen in patients with long-standing gallstones who develop common bile duct obstruction as a result of passage of stones into it. The clinical picture, ultrasonographic findings and laboratory values all suggest that the patient has a common bile duct full of pus. The patient is in septic shock and the key component of management is decompression of the common bile duct. Emergency decompression of the common bile duct with ERCP is usually the first choice and the least risky in a sick patient such as the one in this question.

Elective cholecystectomy will indeed be needed once the acute problem has been resolved. However, if the next step in our planning included only elective surgery, then she would never get it: she would be dead before that. Emergency cholecystectomy will again not deal with the issue of pus in the common bile duct. Emergency surgical exploration of the common bile duct is a procedure that is high risk for such a sick patient because the priority is draining all the pus, which can be achieved with ERCP. Masterly inactivity will kill this patient because acute ascending cholangitis is a potentially lethal diagnosis.

4.16 Carcinoma of the breast   Answers: A B D E

Paget's disease of the nipple presents with redness, itching or eczema of the nipple. Blood-stained nipple discharge may be a feature. There is malignant change within the epithelium of the nipple, which shows 'Paget's cells' and there is associated intraduct carcinoma in 50% of cases.

Breast carcinoma may be hormone dependent. The oestrogen receptor (ER) status forms the basis of endocrine treatment, eg with tamoxifen or aromatase inhibitors such as anastrozole.

Breast-conserving surgery is now increasingly used, ie lumpectomy. Mastectomy is reserved for large tumours, central tumours or for patients who express a preference for mastectomy. Breast reconstruction is also offered to the patient.

4.17 The carcinoid syndrome   Answers: A C E

Carcinoid syndrome presents with:

- flushing
- diarrhoea
- abdominal pain
- bronchospasm
- pulmonary/tricuspid stenosis – late
- hepatomegaly.

Carcinoid tumours are found in the appendix, gastrointestinal tract and lungs. They may secrete 5–hydroxytryptamine (5HT or serotonin) and other hormones. Symptoms are produced by excess 5HT, which is normally metabolised in the liver; symptomatic patients tend to have metastases. Carcinoid of the appendix is usually incidental but can also metastasise to the liver. If the tumour obstructs the appendix it results in appendicitis.

Treatment of carcinoid tumour is by resection. Liver metastases can be embolised or treated with chemotherapy. Octreotide inhibits 5HT release and is used for symptomatic treatment.

4.18 Osteoarthritis of the hip
Answers: C D

Osteoarthritis is a degenerative condition of the joints ('wear and tear') with damage to articular cartilage. It occurs in elderly people, most commonly in the hips and knees and interphalangeal joints. Cartilage-wear damage is increased in load-bearing joints.

Treatment consists of pain relief using analgesics and NSAIDs. Steroids are not beneficial. Mobilisation and weight loss are helpful.

Surgery is indicated in progressive disease when movement is compromised. The joint destruction increases, causing worsening pain and producing deformity. The are following the surgical options:

- Arthrodesis: the joint is fixed in a set position, resulting in a stiff joint, useful only when movement is not required
- Realignment osteotomy: this is used in cases where part of the joint space is intact and weight-bearing surfaces are realigned
- Joint replacement with a prosthesis: this is the treatment of choice in elderly people. Osteoarthritis of the hip requires total hip replacement, not 'knee' replacement – read the question carefully!

Hemiarthroplasty is used in fractures of the neck of the femur, and replaces only half of the articular surfaces.

4.19 Dukes' staging of colorectal cancer
Answers: A B

Dukes' staging of colorectal cancer is made by pathological assessment of the affected bowel and its local lymph nodes. It is therefore not an assessment of distant spread. It is as follows:

A Growth limited to the wall of the colon (ie not through the serosa)
B Extension through the wall and surrounding tissue but not to local lymph nodes
C Metastases in the lymph nodes.

Stage D has been used to describe distant metastases but this was not part of the original classification. In general, staging of carcinoma is useful to predict prognosis and further management, eg chemotherapy, radiotherapy and surgery. In colorectal carcinoma, surgery may be curative for stage A; for stages B and C chemotherapy may be added.

Dukes' staging refers to resected bowel specimens and not to postmortem specimens. The 5-year survival rate after surgery is as follows:

- Dukes' A: 95%
- Dukes' B: 70%
- Dukes' C: 40%.

Note that less than 50% of patients with colorectal cancer are incurable at presentation and therefore do not undergo radical surgery with the aim of cure. These patients die within 5 years.

4.20 Femoral hernia   Answers: A D

A femoral hernia is the passage of peritoneum and its contents (including fat or bowel) into the femoral canal. It is quite likely to become obstructed or strangulated because the femoral canal/ring is narrow. The terms used vary but all have specific meanings, eg:

- Irreducible: cannot be reduced
- Obstructed: luminal contents obstructed but the bowel is viable
- Strangulated: blood supply the bowel is cut off; leads to infarction.

Femoral hernias are more common in women than in men, but in both sexes femoral hernias are less common than inguinal hernias. A femoral hernia arises below and lateral to the pubic tubercle. It is usually small. If it enlarges it tends to be deflected upwards. A cough impulse may not be detectable and therefore it may be difficult to distinguish from a lipoma or an enlarged lymph node.

4.21 Gallstones   Answers: B C E

Gallstones are almost always formed in the gallbladder (by precipitation from bile). They vary in content:

- About 5% are pigment stones
- About 20% are cholesterol stones
- About 75% contain both.

Predisposing factors include high concentrations of bile, stasis and infection. Around 90% of stones are radiolucent. When a stone passes into the duodenum it may be found in the stool. Large stones can pass directly from the gallbladder to the duodenum and cause small bowel obstruction. Chronic inflammation of the gallbladder as a result of gallstones has been implicated in carcinoma of the gallbladder. Gallstones are present in most cases of gallbladder carcinoma. If a stone lodges in the ampulla of Vater it can cause acute pancreatitis. A stone lodged in the common bile duct can cause jaundice, ascending cholangitis or acute pancreatitis.

4.22 Intravenous urography   Answers: A B C E

A ureteric calculus may cause obstruction to urine flow. The urinary tract proximal to the obstruction therefore becomes dilated and swollen. This is visualised by intravenous urography (IVU). For this procedure a 'control' abdominal film (KUB = kidney, ureter and bladder) is taken to look for opacities. Intravenous contrast medium is then injected and further film(s) obtained. Information is obtained about the following:

- Renal size and shape
- Speed of excretion of contrast
- The ureters
- Filling defects/site of obstruction
- The bladder.

In acute obstruction there should be prompt excretion of urine by the unaffected kidney. The unaffected kidney should also be normal in size and shape.

4.23 Burns   Answers: B C D

The estimation of the area of a burn is done by use of the 'rule of nines':

- Head 9%
- Arms 9% each
- Back 18% (2 × 9)
- Front 18% (2 × 9)
- Legs 18% each (2 × 9)
- Palm 1%.

Major burns cause extensive fluid loss and this requires replacement with intravenous colloid and crystalloid. Hypovolaemia, together with haemoconcentration, predispose to thrombosis. The insult to the body causes a stress response and peptic ulceration may result. Another consequence of a major burn is hypothermia, and ice would worsen this.

4.24 Hypotension   Answers: A C D E

Hypotension is a sign of 'shock'. A common cause of this is hypovolaemia, eg as occurs in a gastrointestinal bleed.

Shock is caused by underperfusion of tissues. It is often seen in infarction of the small bowel. Myocardial infarction affects the heart and its function. It may result in a significant decrease in cardiac output. Hypoperfusion results and blood pressure falls.

Gram-negative organisms, eg *Escherichia coli*, are well known for producing exotoxins. These act on the circulation and cause vasodilatation, which results in hypotension.

Intracranial bleeding causes an increase in the intracranial pressure. The effect of this is to decrease heart rate and increase blood pressure (in contrast to hypovolaemia where the cardiovascular response is to increase heart rate and reduce blood pressure).

4.25 Subphrenic abscess   Answers: B C D

A subphrenic abscess occurs as a complication of intra-abdominal infection or surgery. The patient typically develops abdominal pain and a swinging pyrexia with sepsis where no other cause (eg chest or bladder infection) can be found. *E. coli* and *Bacteroides* species are the most common offending organisms.

A subphrenic abscess can occur on the left or right side of the abdomen.

On the right side it occurs between the diaphragm and the liver. It communicates with the peritoneal cavity. Infection here commonly arises from the gallbladder or small bowel perforation. Infection from the right kidney may also result in a right-sided subphrenic abscess.

On the left side it occurs between the diaphragm and left lobe of the liver, with the spleen further to the left. Infection is associated with gastric perforation or is from colon, pancreas or spleen.

Diaphragmatic irritation causes hiccoughs.

Investigations show the following:

- ESR (erythrocyte sedimentation rate): raised
- WCC: raised
- Chest radiograph: pleural effusion occurs on the side of the abscess; empyema may occur
- Ultrasonography and CT: collections are visualised.

The treatment is as follows:

- Drainage: this is the definitive treatment; percutaneous drainage is ultrasonically or CT guided. Antibiotics are also given to prevent sepsis.
- Conservative, with antibiotics only.

Alternatively, surgery may be required.

4.26 Acute appendicitis   Answers: A B E

Acute appendicitis is a very common surgical emergency. The classic symptoms are as follows:

- Pain: this starts as central abdominal pain which shifts to the right iliac fossa

- Anorexia (before pain)
- Nausea and vomiting
- Constipation, but diarrhoea may occur.

The following are the typical signs:

- The patient is flushed; especially in children the tongue is furred, with fetor oris
- There is rebound tenderness and guarding in the right iliac fossa
- Pyrexia (but the patient may be apyrexial) – if the temperature is > 38°C, consider perforation
- Rectal examination may reveal tenderness in the right pelvic area.

The appendix is a vestigial organ attached to the caecum. Usually infection develops in the appendix because it is obstructed by a faecolith.

4.27 Bell's palsy   Answers: A B

Bell's palsy is a lower motor neuron lesion of the seventh cranial nerve, ie the facial nerve, which supplies the muscles of facial expression, sensation to the external auditory meatus, and the salivary and lacrimal glands, and a branch to stapedius. The features are as follows:

- Loss of facial expression on the affected side; there is drooping of the lip and lower eyelid. The patient is unable to smile, whistle or frown. On attempted closure of the eye, the eye tends to roll upwards. The lower eyelid droops and hence complete eye closure is not possible. The patient may require a protective eye patch and lubricant eye drops to keep the eye moist
- Loss of lacrimation
- Loss of taste in the anterior two-thirds of the tongue
- Pain around the ear, caused by inflammation
- Hyperacusis if the nerve to stapedius is affected.

With a lower motor neuron lesion the entire side of the face is paralysed. In an upper motor neuron lesion the upper facial muscles are not affected because occipitofrontalis has a bilateral innervation; so when the patient is asked to raise his or her eyebrows he or she is still able to do so.

The cause of a Bell's palsy is unknown, although there may be a history of a previous viral illness. Treatment is conservative; the symptoms resolve with time. Steroids may be given, but their use is controversial. Around 40% of patients do not fully recover. A seventh nerve lesion associated with herpes zoster virus infection, causing lesions in the external auditory meatus, is known as the Ramsay Hunt syndrome.

4.28 Avascular necrosis Answers: A B C D E

Avascular necrosis is ischaemic necrosis of bone. It is caused by interruption of the blood supply to the bone. It is a well-known complication of the following:

- Trauma, such as fractures, eg of the scaphoid, femoral neck (subcapital), humeral head, lunate and talus, or dislocation, eg of the lunate bone
- Caisson disease
- Infection, eg TB
- Neoplastic lesions
- Metabolic, eg Gaucher's disease
- Connective tissue disease
- Drugs, eg high-dose steroids
- Alcohol abuse
- Vascular disease, eg sickle cell disease
- Idiopathic, eg Perthes' disease.

There is a useful mnemonic for remembering the causes of any condition:

TIN MAN CAN DRIVE

T	**T**rauma
I	**I**nfection
N	**N**eoplasia
M	**M**etabolic
A	**A**utoimmune
N	**N**utritional
C	**C**onnective tissue
A	**A**geing
N	**N**eurological
D	**D**rugs
R	**R**adiotherapy
I	**I**diopathic
V	**V**ascular
E	**E**ndocrine

4.29 Gynaecomastia Answers: B E

Gynaecomastia is a benign condition in which there is enlargement of the breast. This is often unilateral. It is most common in men aged over 50. The causes are as follows:

- Physiological: neonatal or pubertal
- Idiopathic: this is the most common non-physiological cause; it may be unilateral or bilateral
- Chronic liver disease, eg alcoholism, cirrhosis
- Hormones, eg oestrogens; in testicular atrophy hormonal abnormality may occur; hormone-producing tumours, eg testicular cancer
- Drugs, such as oestrogens – diethylstilboestrol (given in prostatic carcinoma), spironolactone, digoxin, cimetidine, steroids, omeprazole, lansoprazole, addictive drugs, such as cocaine. Peptic ulcer disease does not cause gynaecomastia as such, but the drugs used often do.

4.30 Paralytic ileus   Answers: A B D

Causes of paralytic ileus are as follows:

- Laparotomy, ie handling of the bowel prolongs the ileus
- Hypokalaemia
- Peritonitis
- Renal failure, which could cause electrolyte imbalance
- Trauma (eg fracture of a lumbar vertebra)

Calcium is not implicated. Lumbar sympathectomy seems to prevent paralytic ileus.

4.31 In the trauma situation, after an RTA   Answers: A C D

The important screening radiographs in the trauma patient are the cervical spine, chest and pelvis. Further radiographs are directed at areas of interest. Tension pneumothorax is treated by the insertion of a cannula into the second intercostal space (below the second rib), midclavicular line, for immediate release of air. The definitive procedure would then be chest drain insertion.

Bleeding is best controlled by direct pressure if the source is obvious and amenable. In open pneumothorax, an occlusive dressing prevents air being 'sucked' into the chest and expanding the pneumothorax.

Pulse oximetry measures percentage saturation of oxygen in the blood, ie SaO_2 percentage. Arterial blood gas measurements are used to determine PaO_2 (partial pressure of oxygen in the arteries).

4.32 Causes of an acutely painful swelling in the scrotum of an 11-year-old boy   Answers: A B

There are two important descriptive words in this question: first, 'acute' and, second, 'painful'. There are usually few questions on paediatric surgery but it is essential to know the important emergency conditions.

Torsion of the testes requires prompt emergency surgery before ischaemic damage results in necrosis, requiring orchidectomy. It is classically seen in children or adolescents presenting with severe pain of the scrotum, of sudden onset. There may be a history of mild trauma and/or previous episodes of pain. Examination reveals swelling of the scrotum with oedema and a horizontally placed testis. The scrotum is usually exquisitely painful, making palpation of the testicular artery very difficult. The differential diagnosis is epididymo-orchitis. This is a common condition, requiring analgesia and antibiotics; the onset is less acute. Ultrasound examination may be performed to differentiate the two conditions, but is not very successful.

Other causes include:

- trauma
- torsion of a testicular appendage
- strangulated inguinal hernia.

Seminoma usually occurs between 30 and 40 years of age whereas teratoma occurs in a younger age group – 20–30 years.

Varicoceles are varicosities of the veins of the pampiniform plexus. They cause swelling that may disappear on lying down. They are not painful unless thrombosis occurs.

4.33 Intussusception   Answers: B C E

Intussusception is prolapse of the bowel into itself, causing a telescopic effect. It affects the ileum and/or colon, ileocolic being the most common. There may be a focus such as a polyp or carcinoma that forms the apex of the intussusception.

Most instances occur in infants, in whom viral infection causes lymphadenopathy and this may propagate the intussusception. Bowel obstruction may result. Vomiting occurs.

The blood supply to the bowel is compromised. Bleeding may occur, which causes the appearance of what is described as 'redcurrant jelly' on rectal examination. Gangrene of the bowel and peritonitis ensues.

'Twisting' of the bowel is 'volvulus'.

Investigation of intussusception is by barium enema, which is diagnostic as well as therapeutic, the weight of the barium reducing the intussusception. Otherwise, laparotomy is required for minimal reduction of the intussusception or resection of the ischaemic bowel.

4.34 Splenectomy   Answers: A B C D E

Splenomegaly is caused by the following:

- Haematological disease, eg leukaemia, lymphoma, myelofibrosis, polycythaemia rubra vera, spherocytosis, β-thalassaemia
- Infections, eg glandular fever, typhoid, typhus, malaria, schistosomiasis
- Gaucher's disease, amyloid, collagen disease, sepsis
- Cysts, tumours
- Portal hypertension.

Massive splenomegaly is an indication for splenectomy. The following are other indications:

- Rupture after trauma
- Uncontrolled splenic bleeding during colonic surgery (iatrogenic).

The following are the complications of splenectomy:

- Gastric dilatation requiring a nasogastric tube and aspiration
- Thrombocytosis immediately postoperatively. There is a risk of DVT – aspirin should be given
- Sepsis: the spleen clears encapsulated micro-organisms, eg pneumococci (pneumovax), meningococci (meningovax), *Haemophilus influenzae* (give Hib vaccine).

Patients should therefore be given prophylactic immunisation preoperatively. After splenectomy low-dose penicillin is administered daily to prevent overwhelming infection.

In splenectomy for trauma, preoperative immunisation is not possible and the vaccine should be administered a week after splenectomy.

4.35 Gastro-oesophageal reflux   Answers: A B C

Reflux of acid from the stomach into the oesophagus causes oesophagitis. This presents with retrosternal pain, regurgitation and dyspepsia. Bleeding may occur, resulting in iron deficiency anaemia. In chronic oesophagitis, fibrosis occurs, which may result in stricture formation and then presents as dysphagia. Metaplasia of oesophageal epithelium, from squamous to columnar, may occur. This is known as Barrett's oesophagus, which is pre-malignant. Pernicious anaemia is associated with atrophic gastritis, not oesophagitis.

Reflux may be so marked that it causes overspill into the trachea. This is particularly marked at night when the patient lies flat, causing 'nocturnal asthma'; pneumonitis may occur. Other modes of presentation are halitosis and hoarseness of the voice.

4.36 Crohn's disease – radiological features   Answers: B C D

Crohn's disease is investigated with contrast studies:

- Small bowel: a small bowel barium meal and follow-through or small bowel enema
- Large bowel: barium enema.

Radiographs show the following:

- Terminal ileum: irregularity of the mucosa
- Rose-thorn ulcers
- Cobblestone appearance of the mucosa
- Narrowing where there is fibrosis, producing strictures
- Dilatation of the bowel proximal to strictures
- Fistulae.

White cell scans are performed to localise sites of inflammation.

Colonoscopy is often helpful to obtain biopsies. The 'lead-pipe colon' is a feature of ulcerative colitis where there is loss of haustra. Toxic megacolon is a feature of ulcerative colitis.

4.37 Obstructive jaundice   Answers: B D E

The features of obstructive jaundice are:

- icterus
- pain
- malaise
- loss of appetite
- pale stools and dark urine.

A raised bilirubin causes yellow discoloration of the skin and sclera. If a clotting disturbance occurs, bruising may be a feature.

Courvoisier's law states that, in the presence of a painless and palpable gall-bladder, jaundice is unlikely to be the result of stones. (It is more likely to be caused by tumour.) A palpable gallbladder may be a result of stones in the biliary tree or carcinoma causing obstruction.

Stones within the gallbladder tend to cause fibrosis, which results in a shrunken gallbladder that is scarred and therefore unable to dilate.

4.38 Hydrocele   Answers: B C

A hydrocele is a serous collection of fluid within the processus vaginalis. It is idiopathic or results from trauma, infection or neoplasia. The following are the clinical features:

- Scrotal swelling, usually without pain
- The cord is palpable above the swelling
- The testis is not palpable because it is surrounded by fluid
- It is fluctuant
- It is transilluminable
- It is irreducible.

Fertility is not affected.

The treatment is as follows:

- Aspiration (but fluid tends to re-collect)
- Surgical excision.

4.39 Recurrent fistulae   Answers: A B C

Infection in the anorectal region can lead to abscess or fistula formation. The following are the causes of recurrent fistulae:

- Infection (eg TB)
- Crohn's disease (anal fissures are the most common anal lesion)
- Neoplasia
- Ulcerative colitis
- Hidradenitis suppurativa.

Diverticulitis is a common cause of fistulae in the sigmoid colon but not of the anal canal. Remember that a fistula is an abnormal tract connecting two epithelial surfaces.

4.40 Abdominal pain with hypotension   Answers: A D

Abdominal pain radiating to the back and presenting with 'shock' is a leaking abdominal aortic aneurysm until and unless proved otherwise (see Question 1.56, Paper 1).

There is often a history of collapse. The differential diagnosis is:

- acute pancreatitis
- mesenteric thrombosis
- myocardial infarction
- perforated peptic ulcer.

The history, examination and investigations clinch the diagnosis. It is important to make the diagnosis of a leaking abdominal aortic aneurysm promptly because it presents a surgical emergency that requires immediate transfer to theatre. Obtain the following:

- Intravenous access with two large-bore cannulae
- Blood for FBC, U&Es, clotting screen, crossmatch for 10 units of blood.

Resuscitation should maintain blood pressure but avoid overloading with fluids because this would increase the haemorrhage.

The patient requires a central line, urinary catheter and immediate surgery.

Renal colic typically presents with loin pain.

Acute appendicitis causes a localised peritonitis in the right iliac fossa. Shock occurs if the appendix perforates.

Pelvic inflammatory disease is unlikely to cause abdominal pain radiating to the back.

4.41 Buerger's disease   Answers: A B C E

Buerger's disease affects young men who smoke. It affects all limbs. The arteries become obliterated, resulting in ischaemia of the affected areas. The veins and nerves are also affected. Patients present with peripheral ischaemic disease that results in ulcers and digital gangrene. The treatment is to **stop smoking**. Otherwise, progressive ischaemia occurs with gangrene and amputation becomes necessary.

4.42 Anal fissure   Answers: A B D

The treatment of anal fissures may be one of the following:

- Conservative: with laxatives such as lactulose, and local anaesthetic agents, some fissures heal spontaneously.
- Medical: topical vasodilators (glyceryl trinitrate or GTN ointment) can be used to reduce anal spasm, but their use is limited by the side effect of headaches, which can be severe.
- Surgical: this is either by 'anal dilatation' or by 'lateral sphincterotomy'.

Surgery is indicated in cases of persistent fissures that become chronic. At surgery, examination under anaesthesia is performed to exclude other pathology. Rectal examination and sigmoidoscopy are necessary to assess the anorectal canal. When anal fissures are caused by Crohn's disease, sphincterotomy is not advised because there is a risk of sepsis.

4.43 Carpal tunnel syndrome   Answers: C D E

Carpal tunnel syndrome is caused by compression of the median nerve in the carpal tunnel, deep to the flexor retinaculum.

The median nerve supplies the 'LOAF' muscles:

L   lumbricals I and II
O   opponens pollicis
A   abductor pollicis brevis
F   flexor pollicis

These are the muscles of the thenar eminence.

Carpal tunnel syndrome causes wasting of the thenar eminence (the ulnar nerve supplies the muscles of the hypothenar eminence) and weakness of these muscles. Sensory loss occurs in the lateral three and a half fingers. Patients complain of paraesthesia especially in this distribution. There is pain in the forearm that is often worse at night.

On continuous tapping over the flexor retinaculum, the pain may be reproduced – Tinel's sign. Pain may also be reproduced by flexion of the wrist for 1–2 minutes – Phalen's sign.

Application of a tourniquet inflated to greater than arterial pressure may also reproduce the symptoms.

Surgical treatment involves division of the flexor retinaculum.

4.44 Peptic ulcers

Answers: B C E

Peptic ulcers are ulcers of the stomach and duodenum. The emergency complications are haemorrhage, perforation and pyloric stenosis. Haemorrhage is caused by erosion of the mucosa and blood vessel walls.

Perforation occurs when erosion of the bowel goes through the full thickness of the bowel wall.

Chronic ulceration may result in stricture formation caused by fibrosis. This may occur in the body of the stomach, pylorus or duodenum.

Peptic ulcers are associated with the following:

- Cigarette smoking
- Stress
- Genetic factors (eg where there is a family history)
- Hyperparathyroidism: calcium levels are raised which stimulates gastric acid secretion.

Hyperparathyroidism presents with the following:

- Abdominal pain
- Bone disease:
  - subperiosteal erosions visible on radiographs
  - small lytic lesions of the skull (pepperpot skull)
  - cystic lesions of bone
- Renal calculi (ie 'stones, bones and abdominal groans!')
- Drugs, eg aspirin, steroids and NSAIDs
- Post-renal transplantation
- Meckel's diverticulum: may contain ectopic gastric mucosa, which secretes gastrin
- Zollinger–Ellison syndrome.

4.45 Meckel's diverticulum

Answers: B D E

Meckel's diverticulum is present in 2% of the population. It is the embryological remnant of the vitello-intestinal duct, and is situated on the ileum about 2 feet (0.6 m) from the ileocaecal junction. It is not the appendix.

Aide mémoire: RULE OF TWOs – 2% of population, 2 feet from caecum and 2 inches long

It may contain gastrin-secreting mucosa, which stimulates acid secretion by the stomach and results in peptic ulceration.

If a Meckel's diverticulum becomes obstructed it gives rise to inflammation and presents with the features of acute appendicitis. It may become inverted and cause intussusception, which presents as small bowel obstruction.

4.46 Acute extradural haemorrhage   Answers: B C D E

Extradural haemorrhage arises from injury to the middle meningeal artery, causing an extradural collection of blood.

It is usually the result of a head injury, typically producing a 'lucid interval' and then deterioration in conscious level.

Intracranial pressure rises as the bleed is contained within the skull. The clinical features are headache, vomiting, papilloedema, altered conscious level, fits and coma. The localising signs include the following:

- Dilated pupil on the side of the injury
- Hemiparesis
- Hemiplegia.

Blood pressure falls and the heart rate increases in hypovolaemia. Blood pressure rises and the heart rate falls in raised intracranial pressure.

A CT scan is diagnostic and very useful in differentiating between subdural and extradural haemorrhage.

Treatment is by urgent evacuation of the haematoma via a burr hole, or craniotomy and control of the bleeding point.

4.47 Carcinoma of the caecum   Answers: B C

Colorectal carcinoma is common, more than 70% occurring in the distal half of the colon. The sigmoid colon is the most common site. Only about 10% occur in the caecum.

Predisposing conditions are ulcerative colitis, familial adenomatous polyposis (FAP) and hereditary non-polyposis colon cancer (HNPCC).

Right-sided colonic tumours present with microcytic anaemia (iron deficiency), resulting from occult bleeding, a mass in the right iliac fossa and diarrhoea. They rarely cause obstruction. Systemic effects are weight loss, malaise and jaundice/hepatomegaly if liver metastases are present. The treatment for a right-sided tumour is a right hemicolectomy. The treatment for a left-sided tumour is a left hemicolectomy or sigmoid colectomy.

Rectal tumours are treated by anterior resection or abdominal–perineal resection of the rectum. Investigations include the following:

- Barium enema, which may show an obvious lesion
- Colonoscopy: required to visualise caecal tumours and, in addition, has the advantage of obtaining a biopsy. Synchronous tumours can be excluded. Sigmoidoscopy is not sufficient to diagnose caecal lesions. The sigmoidoscope reaches only the splenic flexure

- CT: will demonstrate the tumour, determine liver metastases and allow staging of the disease.

4.48 Paralytic ileus   Answers: A C E

In paralytic ileus, the bowel is quiescent and there is functional obstruction of the bowel. This results in dilatation of the bowel and vomiting. The following are the signs:

- Inspection: abdominal distension
- Palpation: tenderness that may be mild (or even absent)
- Percussion: hyperresonant
- Auscultation: absent bowel sounds.

Paralytic ileus is seen postoperatively, especially when bowel has been handled.

Colicky abdominal pain does not occur because there is no mechanical obstruction and the bowel is not contracting. Radiographs show dilated loops of bowel with gas and fluid levels.

4.49 Dysphagia   Answers: A C D

Dysphagia is difficulty in swallowing. Do not confuse this with dysphasia, which is impaired speech. Dysphagia occurs when there is an obstruction to the passage of solids or fluids in the oesophagus. Obstruction may be in the following positions:

- In the lumen, eg carcinoma of the oesophagus
- In the oesophageal wall, eg benign stricture, carcinoma, pharyngeal pouch, leiomyoma
- Outside the wall, eg carcinoma of the bronchus causing compression
- Resulting from a disorder of motility, eg achalasia, stroke.

4.50 Diverticular disease   Answers: A C D

Diverticular disease is a common condition in western society, caused by lack of fibre in the diet. It is asymptomatic. Inflammation of a diverticulum is 'diverticulitis'. It can occur in the small bowel but is far more common in the colon. It is not associated with malignancy. The complications and their presentations are listed below.

Complication	Presentations
Inflammation	Left iliac fossa pain
Inflammation/haemorrhage	Rectal bleeding
Infection/sepsis/abscess formation	Swinging pyrexia with abdominal pain, sepsis
Perforation	'Rigid abdomen'
Fistulae	Pneumaturia
Stricture formation	Bowel obstruction with distension and vomiting

4.51 Hepatitis B   Answers: B C D

Hepatitis B virus is a DNA virus. It has an incubation period of 2–6 months. It is transmitted in blood products, eg by intravenous drug users or in blood transfusions. Healthcare workers who are at risk of needlestick injuries or other injuries should be immunised with a course of three immunisations. The clinical features include anorexia, malaise, nausea and vomiting. Jaundice and abdominal pain may occur. Liver function is affected and therefore clotting abnormalities may occur. Hepatitis B infection causes chronic hepatitis with an increased risk of cirrhosis and hepatocellular carcinoma.

4.52 Direct hernia   Answers: B C

Inguinal hernias occur above and medial to the pubic tubercle. An indirect inguinal hernia rather than a direct inguinal hernia is controlled (after reduction) by pressure on the internal (deep) ring.

A direct inguinal hernia is caused by weakness of the anterior wall of the inguinal canal so the abdominal contents bulge forward. An indirect inguinal hernia is the passage of abdominal contents along the inguinal canal towards the scrotum. The two can occur together.

A direct inguinal hernia lies medial to the inferior epigastric vessels, whereas an indirect inguinal hernia lies lateral to them.

The risk of strangulation is low in a direct hernia.

4.53 Pancreatitis   Answers: C D

The treatment of pancreatitis depends on the severity of the attack:

- The patient is given intravenous fluids and kept 'nil by mouth'.
- Antibiotics are given if there are signs of infection.
- A nasogastric tube is inserted.
- A urinary catheter is inserted to monitor urine output.
- A central venous pressure (CVP) line may be required to control fluid balance.

- Blood pressure and heart rate are monitored.
- Analgesia is given as required.

For respiratory problems, oxygen is given via a mask; ventilation may be necessary. There is a risk of ARDS.

Surgery is not the treatment of choice in acute pancreatitis.

The clinical picture in acute pancreatitis can be very deceptive.

In chronic pancreatitis, if the pancreatic tissue is severely damaged it is unable to mount a response and therefore a rise in serum amylase does not occur. Hence, a 'normal' amylase level can be seen when there is considerable inflammation.

Other conditions that cause a rise in amylase include perforated peptic ulcer and trauma.

Essentially, the treatment of pancreatitis is conservative. Laparotomy may be required for débridement of severe necrosis as a last resort.

4.54 Carbuncle   Answers: A C D E

A carbuncle is a localised infection of hair follicles and subcutaneous tissue caused by *Staphylococcus aureus*. It affects the adjacent skin and multiple sinuses develop. The back of the neck is a common site. It is more common in people with diabetes, hence the association with glycosuria. Treatment is with flucloxacillin.

4.55 Heparin   Answer: C

Heparin inhibits blood coagulation by inactivation of thrombin and coagulation factors VII, IX, X, XI and XII. Intermittent subcutaneous injection is given for prophylaxis of venous thrombosis (5000 IU twice daily). Intravenous therapy is given for the treatment of DVT, not prophylaxis.

Heparin has a short half-life of about 1 hour. It is reversible with protamine. The best test for monitoring therapy is the activated partial thromboplastin time (APTT).

The INR is a measure of the prothrombin time (PT), which is used to monitor warfarin activity.

Long-term heparin therapy causes osteoporosis, not osteomalacia

4.56 Hyperhidrosis   Answers: D E

Hyperhidrosis is excess sweating of the skin. It is a common complaint and can be very distressing when it occurs in the hands. It classically occurs in young women. The aetiology is unknown but it is thought to be caused by excessive vasomotor activity, via sympathetic nerves. Treatment includes the following:

- Axillary skin excision: the hair-bearing area containing sweat glands is removed as a thin layer of skin
- Cervical sympathectomy: used to abolish palmar sweating; a recognised complication of this is Horner syndrome
- Lumbar sympathectomy: used to abolish sweating of the soles.

4.57 Pseudomembranous colitis   Answers: B C D

Pseudomembranous colitis is colitis caused by antibiotic therapy. Clindamycin was one of the first antibiotics to be implicated but cephalosporin therapy is more common. Pseudomembranous colitis is caused by an overgrowth of *Clostridium difficile*. It causes a profound watery diarrhoea and the formation of a membrane on the intestinal mucosa. Investigation is as follows:

- Sigmoidoscopy and biopsy
- Detection of *C. difficile* toxin in the stool
- Culture of *C. difficile* from the stool.
- *C. difficile* toxin in the serum.

Treatment is oral metronidazole or oral vancomycin.

4.58 Thyroid carcinoma   Answers: A B D

Thyroid carcinoma is divided into four types:

1. Papillary
2. Follicular
3. Anaplastic
4. Medullary.

Papillary carcinoma affects children and young adults, females more than males. It presents as a slow-growing lump. It is slow to spread and does so via the lymphatics. It may therefore present with enlargement of lymph nodes. The thyroid gland moves on swallowing and is not fixed to the skin. There is an association with previous radiation. The standard treatment is total thyroidectomy and the prognosis is excellent.

Follicular carcinoma affects adults aged 40–50 years. It spreads via the bloodstream to lungs and bones, and may therefore present with shortness of breath or bone pain. Treatment is thyroid lobectomy; if metastases are present total thyroidectomy is performed.

Anaplastic tumours present in older patients, aged 60–80 years. It is more common in women than men. Spread is rapid. Patients present with a hard thyroid lump and symptoms of local invasion, such as hoarseness if the recurrent laryngeal nerve is affected or stridor if the trachea is compressed. The prognosis is worse in this type. Surgical treatment is palliative.

Medullary carcinoma is a well-differentiated carcinoma of parafollicular cells, which secrete calcitonin. It affects patients aged 50–70 years. The treatment is total thyroidectomy.

Thyroid carcinomas do not usually cause thyroid dysfunction. Patients are often euthyroid.

4.59 Transplant surgery
Answers: B C D E

Renal transplantation has increased in numbers and success. It is used for patients in chronic renal failure and end-stage renal failure. Consideration is given to the patient's condition; patients over the age of 50 years are not excluded.

Transfer of tissue (eg, skin from one part of the body to another) is an autograft; transfer from person to person is an allograft; transfer from one species to another is a xenograft.

Rejection is a result of the presence of antibodies and is a major problem. Prevention is by tissue typing and immunosuppression.

Any infection must be treated before surgery.

4.60 Amylase
Answers: A C D E

A marked rise in serum amylase occurs in acute pancreatitis (> 1000 IU/L). However, the level is not indicative of severity. The following are other causes:

- Diabetic ketoacidosis
- Perforated peptic ulcer (not > 400 IU/L)
- Acute cholecystitis
- Renal failure
- Strangulated bowel
- The acute abdomen.

Acute appendicitis does not cause raised amylase.

INDEX

The numbers after each entry refer to the paper and question number.

Index

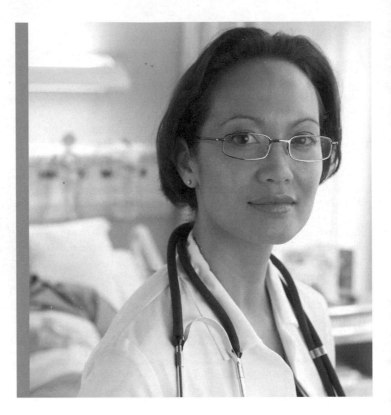

See a specialist

MLP Private Finance plc is part of the MLP Group, one of the leading Independent Financial Advisers in Europe. We specialise in financial planning and wealth management for professionals, and as such our services are tailored to the particular needs of the medical field. MLP provides quality independent advice which means we recommend the most suitable products, plans and funds from the entire marketplace to meet your specific needs and objectives.

We offer financial solutions for: Protection | Insurance | Investments | Savings | Retirement Planning | Mortgages. For more information, contact us on 0845 30 10 999 or info@mlpuk.co.uk or simply visit www.mlp-plc.co.uk.

MLP is the exclusive sponsor of PasTest Undergraduate Finals Revision Courses

MLP Private Finance plc is authorised and regulated by the Financial Services Authority.

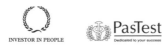

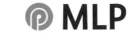